ROCHESTER STORIES

A MED CITY HISTORY

To Nancy—
Enjoy!
Best wishes!

PAUL D. SCANLON, MD

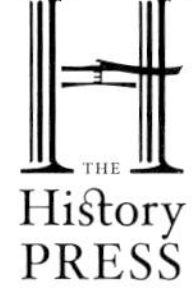

Published by The History Press
Charleston, SC
www.historypress.com

Front cover, bottom: Ear of Corn water tower. *Courtesy of Dean Riggott Photography. Front cover, middle*: Gertrude Booker Granger. *Courtesy of the W. Bruce Fye Center for the History of Medicine, Mayo Clinic, Rochester, Minnesota. Front cover, left and right*: *Author's collection. Back cover*: Aerial of Rochester. *Courtesy of Dean Riggott Photography.*

First published 2021

Manufactured in the United States

ISBN 9781467149167

Library of Congress Control Number: 2021934131

Notice: The information in this book is true and complete to the best of our knowledge. It is offered without guarantee on the part of the author or The History Press. The author and The History Press disclaim all liability in connection with the use of this book.

All who are benefited by community life, especially the physician, owe something to the community.

—Charles Horace Mayo

Contents

Acknowledgements

Writing is generally a solitary activity, but writing a book involves more people than one might expect. During a little more than a year of researching, writing and other tasks, I have crossed paths with quite a few people despite the COVID-19 pandemic.

I would like to thank the staff of the Mayo Clinic W. Bruce Fye Center for the History of Medicine for help with archival materials, including seventeen of the photographs used. This includes Emily Christopherson, Karen Koka, Nicole Babcock and Renee Ziemer. Thanks also to Rosemary Perry in the Section of Publications. Images used are by permission of Mayo Foundation for Medical Education and Research, courtesy of the W. Bruce Fye Center for the History of Medicine, Mayo Clinic, Rochester, Minnesota. Two of the images are also by permission of Mayo Foundation for Medical Education and Research but courtesy of Mayo Clinic Media Support Services.

Thanks to my good friend Dean Riggott, of Dean Riggott Photography, for a generous selection of gorgeous photographs. Thanks to Krista Lewis, Wayne Gannaway and Dana Knaak at the History Center of Olmsted County for photographs, archival information and encouragement. Thanks to Jeff Pieters and Ken Klotzbach at the *Post Bulletin* for photographs and research help. And thanks to Mark Harry, Jacob Brettin, Jodi Jacobson, Christie's, the National Audubon Society and the Minnesota Geologic Survey for photographs and other images.

Thanks to the Honorable Kevin A. Lund for amazing youth mentorship, historic preservation and community leadership and for singlehandedly saving Northrop School. Thanks to John Kruesel, Stevenson Williams and Jane Bisel for providing a badly needed conscience for historic preservation in Rochester.

All postcard images are scanned from my personal collection. To avoid copyright encroachment, all postcard images are either in public domain because of age (pre-1923) or are uncopyrighted images (no photographer identified). Other historical images, maps and photographs, unless noted otherwise, are from my personal collection, all rights reserved.

Thanks to my friends, colleagues and role models as historical writers: Anthony J. (Tony) Bianco III; W. Bruce Fye, MD; and Christopher J. Boes, MD (though I do not pretend to have their level of professionalism or academic rigor as a writer or historian). Thanks also to others who have written useful and relevant books of local history, including Amy Jo Hahn, Virginia Wright-Peterson, Ken Allsen, Ted St. Mane, Judith Hartzell, Harriet Hodgson, the late Harold Severson and Mearl Raygor and my dear friend the late Alan Calavano. And thanks to numerous *Post Bulletin* writers over the years, particularly Tom Weber.

Thanks to John Rodrigue and Hayley Behal, my editors, and to their colleagues at The History Press, for all their professionalism and skillful production.

Thanks to my former colleagues in the Division of Pulmonary and Critical Care Medicine, the Dolores Jean Lavins Center for Humanities in Medicine and the Mayo Clinic as a whole for flawlessly shouldering my former workload as I moved into retirement.

Thanks and lots of love to my wife, Maggie; Brian and Marianne; Luke; Kelsey and Jake; the grandkids, Will, Charlie, Tommy, Kinley, Ben, Liam and Idris; my mom, Jane; and my sister, Patricia, and her husband, Harrison. They provided support, encouragement and inspiration to me through this surprisingly pleasant though lengthy process. I would also like to remember my grandfathers, Maurice and Edwin; my dad, Paul W.; and my brother, Barry, who provided a lot of memories.

Preface

Historical but Not a Conventional History

This book is prompted by a family tradition of storytelling. My paternal grandfather, Maurice Scanlon, was descended from Irish immigrants. James Scanlon and his wife, Ellen, née Tangney, both born in 1823 in County Kerry, immigrated to Massachusetts, where they were married in 1850 and settled in upstate New York. Their grandson Maurice Daniel was born on a farm outside of Fulton, New York, on Christmas Eve 1890, the seventh of eleven children.

Maurice was a wonderful storyteller. Having grown up on the family farm, Maurice traveled west as a young man. He boxed professionally in Detroit and worked as a stevedore in San Pedro Harbor in Los Angeles. During the Great War (World War I), he returned to manage the family farm with his nearly sixty-year-old father. Near the end of the war, he married Mary "May" Warmke. During Prohibition, he made a side income by selling hard cider and bathtub gin, always provided gratis to the local constabulary, who never bothered his business otherwise. After Prohibition, he sold the family farm and moved into town to a house that was paid for with proceeds from bootlegging. He then served on the Fulton, New York Police Department for a lengthy career, retiring at the age of sixty-five. He was reputedly a tough cop with a nickname of "Balls" Scanlon. As a retiring police officer in 1955, he bought into Social Security for a one-time payment of $300 and received benefits in addition to his police pension until he died at age ninety-six. He was a fur trapper as a youth, and in retirement, he had a business buying furs from local trappers (mostly muskrat and raccoon with

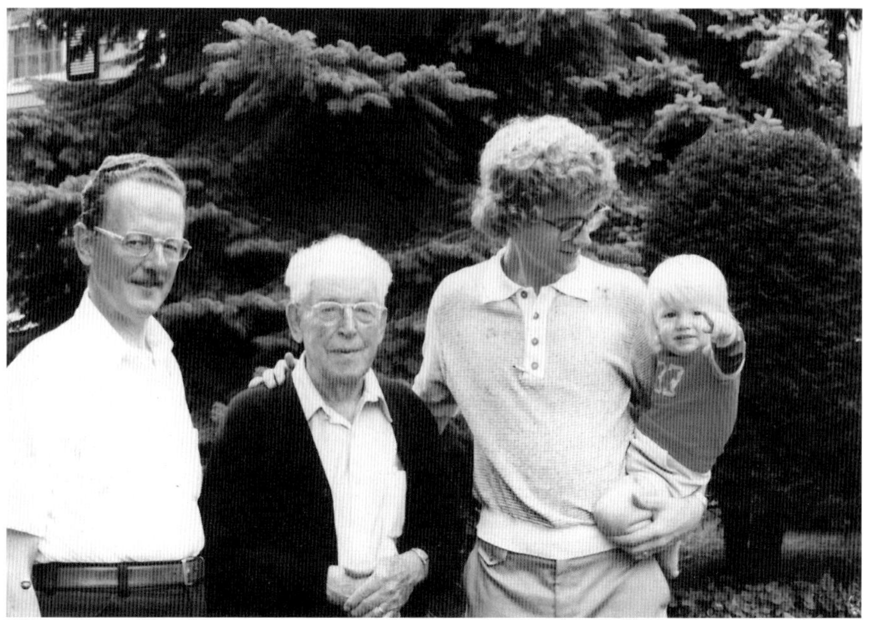

Four generations of Scanlons—Paul W., Maurice, Paul D. and Luke, summer 1980.

occasional fox, mink, skunk and pine marten), which he then sold to the Hudson's Bay Company. He always kept a pint of inexpensive whisky by the kitchen table for visiting trappers and friends. He called it "trappers' bait." He also raised chickens and participated in cockfighting long after it was outlawed. He was well into his eighties when he was arrested for the last time at a cockfight in Pennsylvania. He always carried his police badge for such occasions. Needless to say, he had some stories to tell. Family members always said, "We should write these down," but they never did. It's been one of my regrets as an adult that my grandfather's stories were not preserved. I had some of the same thoughts regarding my own nuclear family with our sometimes-hilarious missteps and misdeeds, which might be worthy of preservation, at least for reference in the family.

A parallel thought popped up about Rochester. It is an interesting town, the home of the best and one of the largest medical centers in the world. There are many resources and references about Rochester, but no comprehensive history has been written, and it's been 111 years since Joseph A. Leonard's *History of Olmsted County* was published. Mearl Raygor's *The Rochester Story*, from 1976, is a nice brief summary but is now 45 years out of date. Harold Severson's *Rochester: Mecca for Millions* was published in 1979.

Harriet Hodgson's *Rochester: City of the Prairie* was published in 1989. It gives summary histories of many local businesses. All are out of print but available from online book dealers. Several more recent books provide some history, mostly related to buildings (Ted St. Mane, *Rochester, Minnesota*, 2003; Alan Calavano, *Postcard History Series: Rochester*, 2008; Amy Jo Hahn, *Lost Rochester*, 2017; Dean Riggott, *Rochester, Minnesota: A Visual and Historic Journey*, 2012; and Ken Allsen, *Houses on the Hill: The Life and Architecture of Harold Crawford*, 2003; *A Century of Elegance: Ellerbe Residential Design in Rochester, Minnesota*, 2009; and *Old College Street*, 2012).

As a native of Rochester and son of a Mayo Clinic physician, I have memories of Mayo Clinic and Rochester events that parallel the memories of people twenty or thirty years my senior. With an interest in the histories of Mayo Clinic and Rochester, I am frequently asked to tell many of these stories to friends, colleagues and visitors.

Although most people like stories, many of the same people think that history is boring. A problem with the structure of most history books is that they must be read continuously and completely from front to back. Extracting a particular story line can be complex and stretched out through the book. Readers' areas of interest and desire for detail vary, so writing a history with just the right amount of detail is problematic. Lacking a comprehensive history of Rochester, it occurred to me that the most utilitarian approach to telling people about Rochester would be to simply tell the stories. Rather than a linear comprehensive history from beginning to end, a series of point-by-point stories, each succinct and self-contained, readable in a few minutes, might be more helpful. Many can be told in response to a question, such as the most obvious and frequently asked: Why did they build the Mayo Clinic out here, in "fly-over country," in the cornfields? Other questions include: What happened to the local Native Americans? What is the origin of the name Zumbro? Why all the hotels? What about the Falcons? Subway? You're kidding, right? Needless to say, the number of possibilities is nearly endless, so selection has been a matter of choice among the stories I know well enough to tell or write about. Word limits are strict, so there are a lot more stories that I could have told instead. The table of contents presents the organization in roughly chronological order. The stories can be read in that order but stand independently and can be read in any order or individually.

I am not a professional historian and have neither the training nor the desire to produce a formal history of Mayo Clinic. Happily, that task has been taken up by my good friend Anthony J. Bianco III. His work is nearly complete, and I eagerly await the fruits of his years of careful research. I

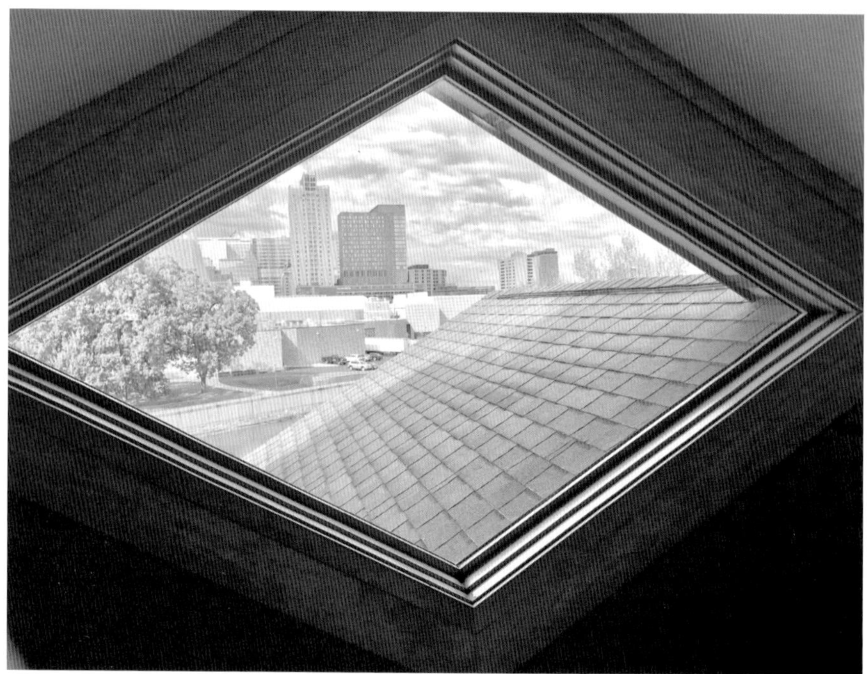

In my view. Downtown Rochester from my attic. *Courtesy of Mark Jay Harry.*

also do not wish to duplicate the work of others. The architectural history of Rochester, with descriptions of buildings and their histories, has been addressed in different ways by the authors above, so I have not attempted to repeat their work. When I write of a building or tell something related to Mayo Clinic, it is generally to tell a story from a different perspective.

Thus, this is historical but not a history in the usual sense. Some of the resources are scarce, including the histories of Olmsted County of 1866 (imagine writing a history of a place that is only eleven years old!), 1883 and 1910, as well as A.T. Andreas's *Historical Atlas of the State of Minnesota* of 1874. As a collector of historical artifacts, I have managed to acquire these and other resources. A variety of online resources have been helpful, particularly the *Post Bulletin*, the local newspaper. The archives of the History Center of Olmsted County and the archives of the Mayo Clinic in the W. Bruce Fye Center for the History of Medicine have been very helpful resources as well (see Sources, page 201).

1
Small-Town Beginnings

Why Rochester? 1854

The first English-speaking settlers arrived in Rochester in the spring and summer of 1854. Four groups of people claimed priority. One of the first two groups to arrive was a crowd of government surveyors led by Thomas Simpson. From the location of the village of Simpson (eight miles to the southeast), they could see mists arising from falls to the northwest. They traveled to the Zumbro River, crossing by what is now Fourth Street Southeast near Broadway. They attempted to make a land claim by constructing a small crude shack on the site. They subsequently realized that as government employees, they were not eligible to make a land claim.

A different group, consisting of E.S. Smith, Charles Eaton and Wheeler Sargeant, came from Winona, arriving in mid-March. Some say they were first, while others say that they "jumped" the claim by Simpson's group, destroying the shack and removing evidence of the prior claim. They made their claim at what is now First Avenue Southwest, south of Fourth Street, and built their own shack as evidence of their claim.

Meanwhile, Thomas Cummings and Robert McReady and his family arrived in the late spring or early summer and established claims a mile to the west, with Cummings claiming what is now the Kutzky neighborhood (west of downtown) and McReady claiming the quarter section (160 acres) to the north of that.

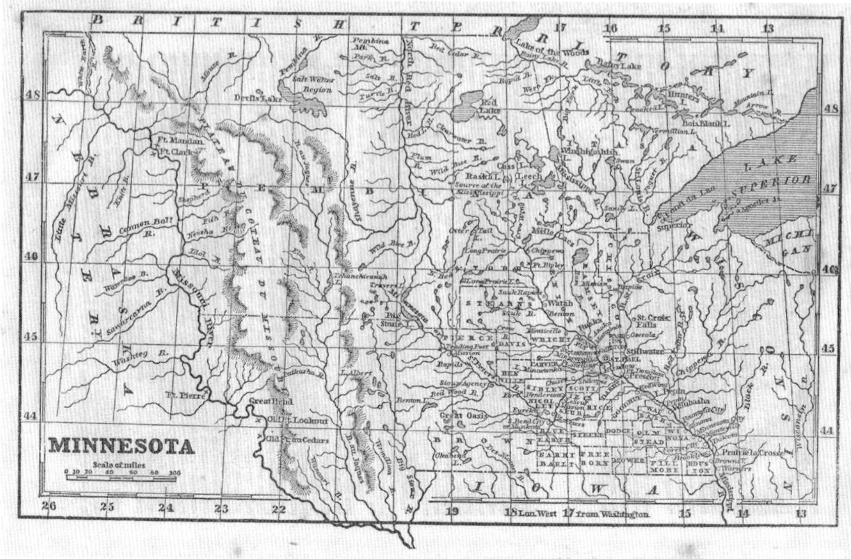

Map of Minnesota Territory, circa 1855. *Source unknown.*

Finally, on July 12, George Head, traveling with his father and his brother, arrived from Wisconsin. The Head group jumped the claim of the Winona group and began to tear down their shack. Smith and Eaton confronted the Heads. They were armed and threatened violence. The dispute was ultimately settled nonviolently, with a payment by Head to members of the Winona group, leaving Head with a valid claim but not the first claim, which is credited to Cummings and McReady.[1]

Head was acquisitive of land claims, and several were questionable at best. Despite his ethics, he is generally regarded as the "Father of Rochester." He named Rochester, making Minnesota one of seventeen states with a town by that name. Ohio and New York each have two towns named Rochester. Joseph A. Leonard wrote:

> *George Head told me that he named the town Rochester because the falls, or, rather, rapids, reminded him of the water power at Rochester, New York, where he once lived. No one who knew him would suspect George of being of a poetic temperament; but what an imagination must have been his to find any resemblance between the gentle purling rapids below College Street bridge, mere ripples on the surface of a quiet little stream, and the majestic cataracts, with their falls of twenty, seventy and ninety-five feet, that furnish the unlimited power of New York's great manufacturing city!*[2]

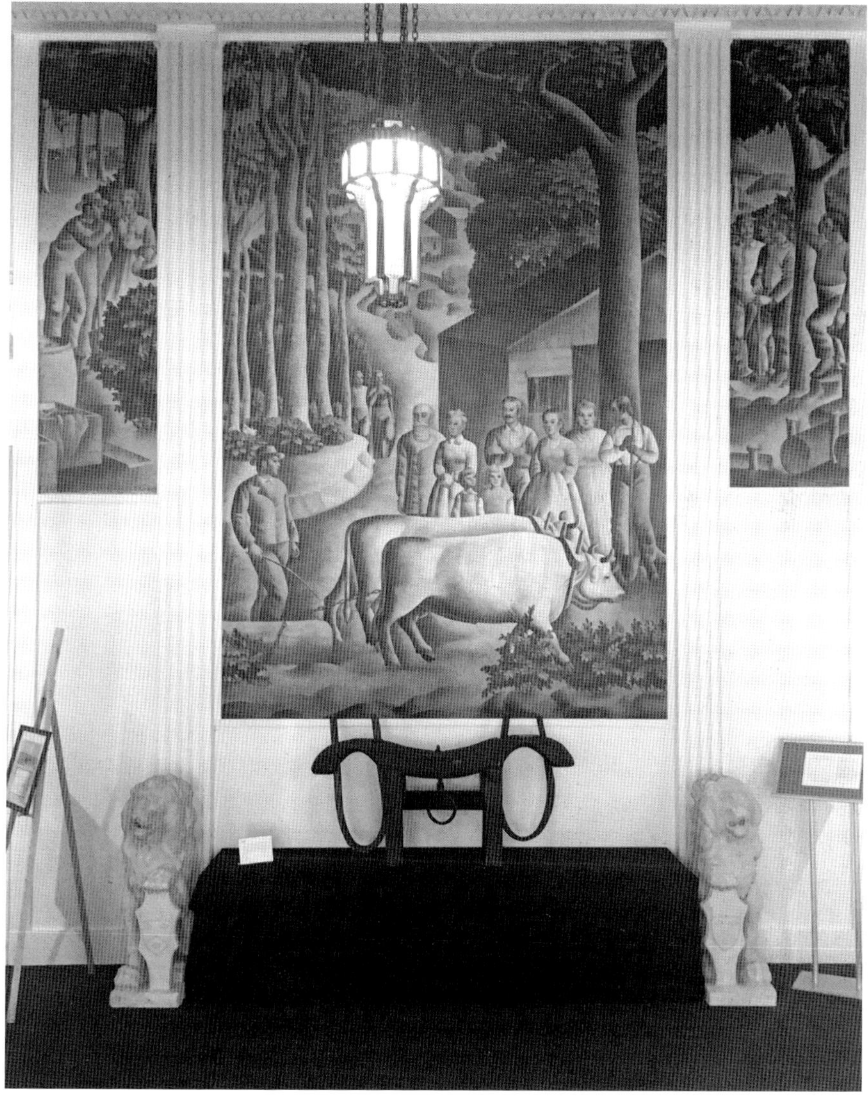

Mural of George Head with oxen. *Courtesy of the History Center of Olmsted County, photo by Paul D. Scanlon (PDS).*

Head also supposedly named and created Broadway by dragging a log behind a team of oxen the length of the road, with his wife following behind on a horse to inaugurate the new thoroughfare. That scene is shown (minus his wife) in a Depression-era mural from the old post office, which was preserved and is on display at the History Center of Olmsted County.

Head's home at the foot of Broadway became an inn and tavern, which he managed until he sold it after a few years. He was very successful for a time, but his business eventually failed, and he moved to Fergus Falls in 1873. He died in Bermuda in 1883 and is buried at Oakwood Cemetery.

The first grocer in Rochester was Hugh Mair. He bought a log structure built by J.D. Jenkins in 1855. Included in Mair's stock was a cask of liquor, the first brought to Rochester, which he sold by the drink. W.H. Mitchell claimed that "the cask was never allowed to get empty, so long as there was plenty of water in the Zumbro....When cold weather came on, the whiskey froze so hard that it had to be sold in chunks, and thawed by the fire, before it could be drank."[3] Leonard told the same story and concluded, "It was a common joke that Mair sold whisky by the pound."[4]

The first brick building in Rochester was erected by L.H. Kelly in 1858 at the northeast corner of Broadway and College Streets (Fourth Street South). It is still standing and contains the central reference survey marker from which all surveys in the city derive. It served for many years as Powderly's Boot Shop. In recent years, it housed Huey's Cigar Store, then Gretchen MacCarty Designs and most recently law offices, first for Kevin Lund and then the Patterson Firm.

IS OLMSTED SPELLED CORRECTLY?

Olmsted (no *a*) County was incorporated in 1855, while Minnesota was still a territory. It was named in honor of David Olmsted, who never lived here. He was born in Fairfax, Vermont, in 1822. He was an Indian trader for eight years among the Ho-Chunk (Winnebago) in Iowa before coming to Minnesota in 1848. He served as president of the first Minnesota Territorial Council in 1849 and owned and edited the *Minnesota Democrat*. He settled in St. Paul in 1853 and was elected the first mayor of St. Paul in 1854. After serving one term, he was replaced by Alexander Ramsey. He then moved to Cuba because of failing health but did not recover. He died at his mother's home in Vermont in 1861 at the age of thirty-eight.[5]

David Olmsted is sometimes confused with Fredrick Law Olmsted, who was born nine days earlier in Hartford, Connecticut, and became a famous landscape architect, journalist and social commentator who designed Central Park in New York. I found no indication that the two were related.

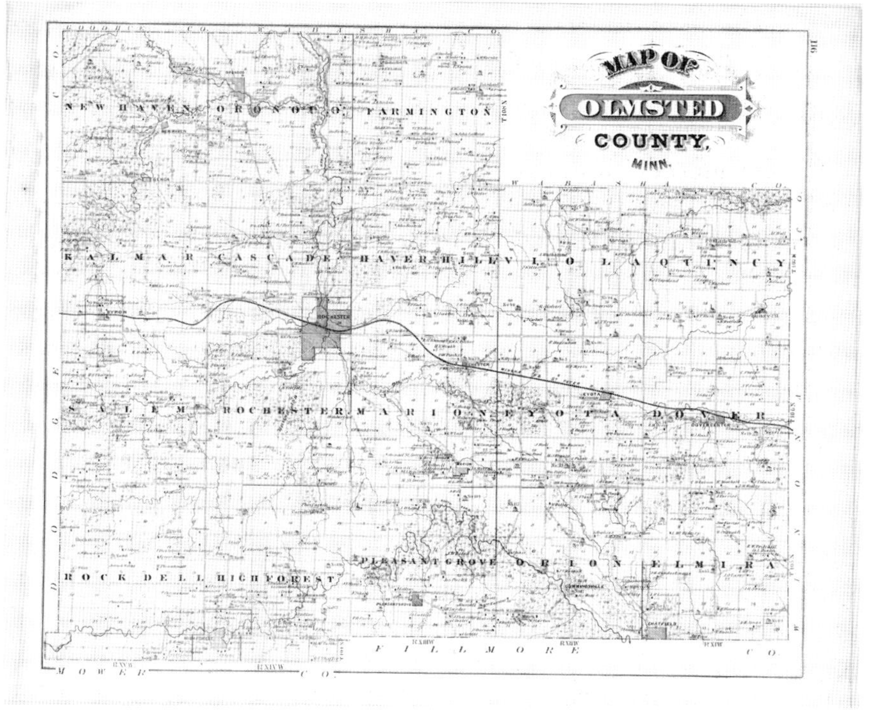

Map of Olmsted County. *From Andreas's* Historical Atlas of the State of Minnesota, *1874.*

Rochester sits in the center of Olmsted County and seems a logical choice for the county seat; however, Oronoco has the greatest potential for waterpower in the county and rivaled Rochester in the early days, as did the village of Marion. The location of the county seat of Olmsted County was decided by popular vote in the spring of 1857. Marion and Oronoco had populations nearly equal to Rochester. When the votes were counted, Marion received the most votes. It was noted, however, that the number of votes from both Marion and Rochester exceeded their populations. Rochester contested the vote. When the legitimate vote was tallied, Rochester was declared the county seat.

A minor gold rush occurred in the fall of 1858 along the Zumbro in downtown Rochester and also below Oronoco. Several small gold nuggets were found, and mining operations in both locations yielded minimal amounts of gold flake. Production was not economically viable, and efforts were terminated in June 1859 after the second of two seasonal floods wiped out the mining facility in Oronoco.

Histories of Olmsted County and Other Sources

Three comprehensive histories of Olmsted County have been written. The first was by W.H. Mitchell in 1866, titled *Geographical and Statistical History of the County of Olmsted, Together with a General View of the State of Minnesota, from Its Earliest Settlement to the Present Time*. Imagine writing a history of a county when it's only eleven years old. Barely a pamphlet, it contains 118 pages of text and measures 4½ by 6¾ inches. It is out of print and exceedingly rare but has interesting insights and details.

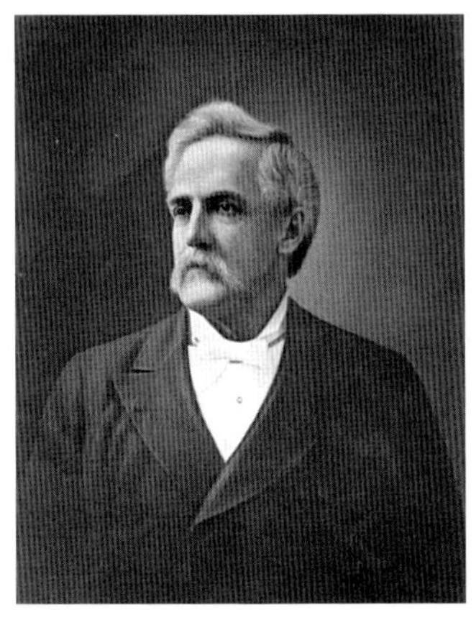

Honorable Joseph A. Leonard. *From frontispiece of* History of Olmsted County, Minnesota, *1910.*

The second history, from 1883, includes Winona and Olmsted Counties, with pages 617 to 1,148 devoted to Olmsted County. The latter portion was written primarily by Samuel William Eaton, as indicated by the introduction to the section on Olmsted County, with other contributors acknowledged. Eaton, like Mitchell and Leonard, was a newspaper editor and publisher, judge and elected politician. His history is well organized and extraordinarily detailed, particularly with regard to education finance and administration, judicial proceedings, geology and the descriptions of the devastation from the tornadoes of 1883.

The third is the best known, *History of Olmsted County, Minnesota* by Honorable Joseph A. Leonard, from 1910. It contains a total of 674 pages, of which the first 297 were written by Leonard with great detail and personal commentary, though a rather rambling chronology. The remaining 377 pages of Leonard's history (and the final 240 pages of the 1883 Winona/Olmsted history) are anonymously authored biographies of Olmsted County settlers and prominent citizens. Leonard cites both Mitchell's and Eaton's histories; they knew each other. Leonard was a physician, lawyer, judge, Civil War veteran major and newspaper owner and editor who lived in Rochester from 1858 until his death in 1908 at the age of seventy-eight. In his late years he served as U.S. consul to Leith, Scotland; Calcutta, India; and Shanghai, China, sequentially. He spent his last five years in retirement compiling his history, which was published posthumously. All three histories are rare in their original editions, but all three are available as reprinted by the Higginson Book Company of Salem, Massachusetts. I have relied on original editions of the first and third but a reprint of the 1883 history.

The Zumbro River (The Mighty Z)

I used to assume that the names *Zumbro* and *Zumbrota* were Native American in origin. They are not. In the language of the local Natives, Dakota, the river is called Waziouja, which translates as "hindered river." The name of the nearby village of Wasioja derives from the river, which flows through it (the South Branch of the Middle Fork). French-speaking traders and trappers, who traveled through this region for a century and a half before English-speaking settlers arrived, translated the Dakota name and called it Riviere des Embarras, which means "river of obstructions." If you paddle the Zumbro River, it has a tortuous course with many turns obstructed by dead trees ("snags") washed out by spring floods. It is challenging to navigate in a canoe. When English-speaking settlers arrived in the 1850s, the French name sounded to them like "River de Zumbra," hence the name, which on early maps is variously spelled as Zumbro, Zumbra, Zambro, Ambras and Embarrass.[6]

It seems like the river is everywhere around Rochester. If one travels on Highway 52 from south of Rochester to north of Zumbrota (25 miles), one crosses the river four times, each section running west to east. The crossings include: 1) the South Fork, just south of Apache Mall; 2) the South Branch of the Middle Fork at Lake Shady by Oronoco; 3) the North Branch of the Middle Fork, also at Lake Shady; and 4) the North Fork just north of Zumbrota. The two branches of the Middle Fork converge at Lake Shady and then meet up with the South Fork east of Oronoco at the upper end of Lake Zumbro. The North Fork joins the rest a few miles north of the power dam at Lake Zumbro. Canoeing on the Zumbro is very scenic, with abundant wildlife, particularly eagles, blue heron, kingfishers and wood ducks, as well as deer, raccoons, beavers and turtles. Travel from Rochester to the Mississippi is 81 miles by water, with only one portage at the power dam. If you are observant, you can see a variety of beautiful native mussel shells with interesting names, such as giant floaters, ellipses, black sandshells, lilliputs, muckets, creepers, fatmuckets, deertoes, cylindrical and fragile

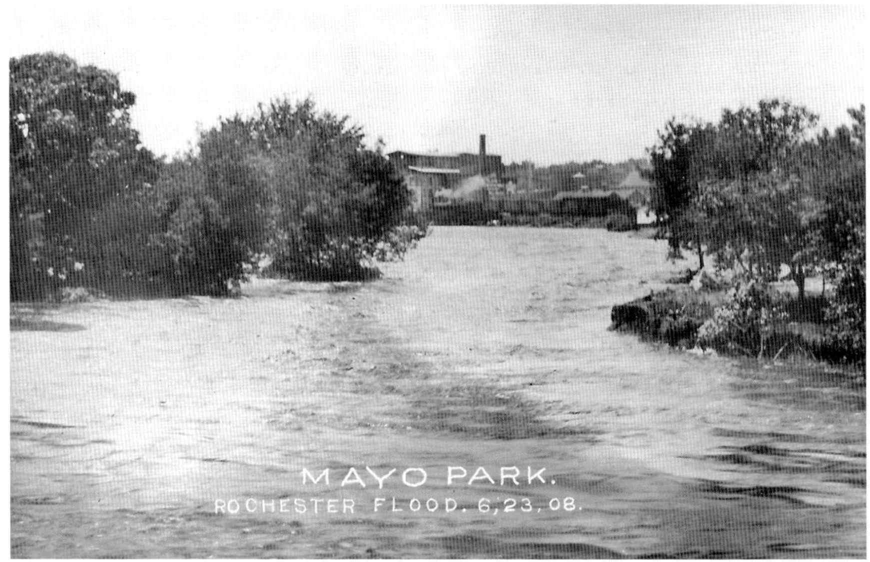

Postcard of Zumbro flood, 1908, with Mayo Park on right and Olds & Fishback Mill in the distance.

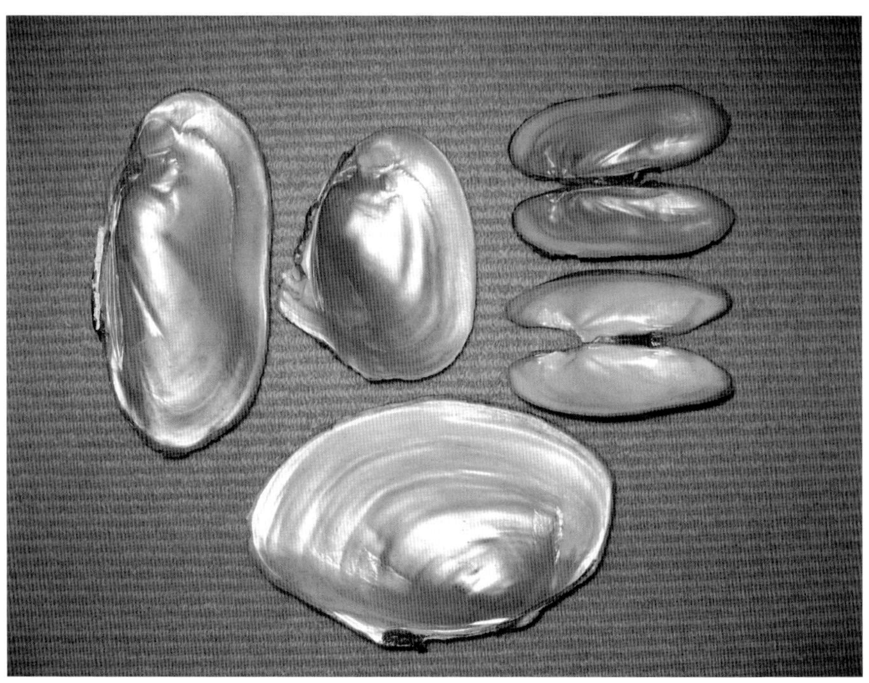

Lake Zumbro mussels. (*Clockwise from upper left*): black sandshell, pink heelsplitter, black sandshell, creeper and giant floater. *Photo by PDS.*

papershells, plain pocketbooks, threeridges, flutedshells, round pigtoes and white, creek and pink heel-splitters. (A fishing license is required to collect, and taking live specimens or listed species is not permitted.)[7] The Zumbro flows through the Richard J. Dorer State Forest, the largest state forest in Minnesota (1,016,227 acres or 1,588 square miles). There are numerous places where the nearest road is half a mile away, so it can be a very solitary experience, sometimes more so than in the Boundary Waters Canoe Area in northern Minnesota.

People who do not know the Zumbro sometimes disdainfully call it the "Scumbro." Through the city, the river is often silty and turbid, primarily because of runoff from construction sites in the city and careless riverbank management in agricultural areas. Strict regulations apply to both, but enforcement is lax. As the river flows north from Rochester, the natural meandering results in settlement of the particulates, gradually clearing it of the mire of civilization. The clearest water in the river is just downstream (north) from the power dam at Lake Zumbro. The bottom is readily visible to a depth of four to five feet or deeper. Interestingly, that spot is the home of an introduced population of muskellunge, as well as huge carp. I like to remind the disrespectful that in the absence of humanity, the river was pristine for millions of years before us, as it will be for millions of years after we are gone.

What Happened to the Local Indians? 1862

The population of North and South America in 1492 has been estimated as high as 50 to 100 million indigenous people.[8] That population was reduced by 80 to 90 percent by infectious diseases imported by European immigrants (smallpox, measles, influenza, typhus, bubonic plague, cholera, typhoid, tuberculosis and others), plus four hundred years of genocide by the governments and armies of white immigrants. The massacres at Sand Creek in Colorado in 1864 and Wounded Knee, North Dakota, in 1890 are two of many examples of U.S. government treatment of indigenous people.

In 1679, Daniel Greysolon, called Le Sieur du Lhut, reached the area of Duluth via Lake Superior. The city of Duluth was named after him, with some creative spelling. He lived and traded among the Ojibwe and Dakota and explored as far as Lake Mille Lacs and the headwaters of the Mississippi near the location of Bemidji. The following year, 1680, French-speaking fur traders, accompanied by Father Louis Hennepin, traveled upriver on the Mississippi as far as St. Anthony Falls in what is now downtown Minneapolis. Many years later, in 1820, Fort Snelling was established overlooking the convergence of the Minnesota and Mississippi Rivers. In 1825, the peace treaty was signed between the Ojibwe and the Dakota at Prairie du Chien. Northern Wisconsin and northern Minnesota were controlled by the Ojibwe (also called Chippewa or Saulteaux or Sauteur). West central Wisconsin and Minnesota south of Fort Snelling, extending out to the upper Missouri Valley, was controlled by the Dakota, also called Sioux. In the 1851 Treaties of Traverse de Sioux (signed by the Sisseton and Wahpenton) and Mendota (signed by the Mdewakanton and Wahpekute bands), the Eastern Dakota (also called Santee or Isanti) ceded twenty-four million acres (thirty-seven thousand square miles) of their land for white settlement and agreed to relocate to a much smaller region along the Minnesota River west of Mankato. In exchange, they were to receive regular payments and supplies. They were forced to give up a portion of their reservation in 1858.[9]

Rochester was first settled by English-speaking settlers in 1854 and was incorporated in 1858. There was no settlement of Native Americans in Rochester, the closest being in Oronoco. Before the treaty, the Eastern Dakota were primarily nomadic but had settlements along the Mississippi near what are now La Crosse, Winona, Wabasha and Red Wing. This group was sometimes called Wapasha, after a series of chiefs of the eighteenth and nineteenth centuries. The land between the Mississippi and Mankato was migratory hunting grounds for the Dakota. The Mississippi settlements and lands to the west were vacated according to terms of the treaty. Other tribes of Dakota and related Lakota were farther west, mainly in the Dakota Territory that subsequently became the states of North and South Dakota, as well as northwest Iowa and northeast Nebraska. At the beginning of white settlement, Eaton notes that "Indians were quite numerous but peaceable."[10] But soon interactions dwindled, with only a few documented instances of indigenous people camping in or traveling through Olmsted County.

Two locations where Natives were frequently seen at first were near Oronoco and in Salem Township. Eaton says of Oronoco: "The Indians were very numerous in this locality during the early days, and often encamped in large numbers on the banks of the river a mile below the village....The pioneers were surrounded by Indians a good deal of the time, but never suffered any serious annoyances from them."[11] Leonard says of the Natives near Oronoco: "Small parties of Chippewa and Sioux Indians were frequently camped about the village in its earliest days, and

Mrs. Hodges remembers a camp of two or three hundred the first season—probably attracted by the good fishing. They were perfectly friendly."[12] Mitchell described the Salem interactions:

> *During the winter of 1854–5, the Indians, in passing through the town, on their way from one belt of timber to another, made Mr. Hurd's house a regular stopping place.* [Hurd was the first settler of Salem Township.] *From twenty to twenty-five would sometimes come into his small house at a time and ask and even demand whatever they wanted, and Mr. Hurd with a frank generosity, never let them go away empty-handed, but satisfied all of their wants. They never molested anyone, but being hungry they demanded the means to satisfy the cravings of their appetites.*[13]

In the fall of 1854, a group of about two hundred Dakota camped in what is now Silver Lake Park. They suffered an outbreak of smallpox or a similar illness, resulting in the death of four of their party. Two more died during the winter, one of the same disease and one of an injury. The deceased were buried above ground in traditional graves in what is now Indian Heights Park on an eastern promontory overlooking the Zumbro River. (Silver Lake had not yet been built.) Those graves were thought to have been obliterated by the tornado in 1883.[14] No evidence of their existence has been found since then (despite generations of children looking). The precise location of the graves is not known and might have been excavated for the construction of the Crenlo plant. After staying in their first location for six weeks, the encamped group moved twice during the winter, first to Bamber Valley and later to the north end of town. In the spring, they left, and the Dakota were not seen thereafter in Olmsted County. For up to eight years afterward, small groups of Ho-Chunk (or Winnebago) would occasionally be seen traveling from their Minnesota reservation to visit their former home in Wisconsin. A small group of Ho-Chunk camped briefly near West Second Street in 1862.[15]

The Dakota War of 1862 occurred during the early stages of the Civil War. Payments that were promised to the Dakota by treaty were chronically delayed, and the Natives were systematically cheated of most of their payments by the agents. On August 15, in frustration at this treatment, a contingent of the Mdewakanton and Wahpekute Dakota met with the agents at the Lower Sioux Agency near Redwood Falls, demanding their payments. They were on the verge of starvation as a result of a poor harvest and requested sale of food on credit in anticipation of the payments. A trader named Andrew Myrick reportedly said, in the Natives' presence: "As far as I am concerned, if they are hungry, let them eat grass." On August 17, four young Dakota men, frustrated after an unsuccessful hunt, killed five white settlers. The next day, a larger group of warriors attacked the Lower Sioux Agency and burned it. Among those killed, Andrew Myrick was found dead with his mouth stuffed with grass. The same day, Natives attacked a militia force in the Battle of Redwood Ferry and killed twenty-four soldiers, including Captain John Marsh. Other Dakota groups attacked white settlements along the Minnesota River Valley, including Milford, Leavenworth and Sacred Heart, destroying the villages and killing many settlers. Ironically, the cash for the treaty payments was delivered to the agency on August 19, the day after it was attacked, too late to interrupt the evolving disaster.

The Dakota continued their offensive by attacking the settlement of New Ulm on August 19 and again on August 23. They burned part of the town, but the residents defended the town from being overrun. The Dakota attacked Fort Ridgely on August 20 and 22 (on the river between Redwood Falls and New Ulm). They were not able to take the fort, but they ambushed a relief party traveling from the fort to New Ulm on August 21. Dr. William Worrall Mayo, the father of the Mayo brothers, was an active participant in the Battle of New Ulm, both as a combatant during the battle and in the care of the wounded, both white and Native, during and after the battle.

The Minnesota militia was brought in to assist the locals. On September 2, they suffered a defeat by the Natives at the Battle of Birch Coulee, sixteen miles from Fort Ridgely. An exploratory party of militia was attacked by the Dakota. Thirteen soldiers were killed and forty-seven wounded, compared with only two Dakota killed. Throughout this time, attacks continued in the Minnesota River Valley and extending westward into the Dakota Territory, near Fort Snelling and St. Cloud, and north along the Red River of the North as far as Fort Garry (near Winnipeg, Manitoba). Alarm spread throughout the region. Tens of thousands of settlers evacuated from twenty-three counties. A year later, nineteen counties remained evacuated.[16]

On September 6, President Lincoln appointed the Department of the Northwest, consisting of several Minnesota Volunteer Infantry Regiments, ordered to "quell the violence" under the command of General John Pope. Pope had recently suffered a humiliating defeat at the Second Battle of Bull Run, after which he was relieved of his command. He declared his intent "utterly to exterminate the Sioux....They are to be treated as maniacs or wild beasts."[17] Thanks to its artillery, the army won a decisive victory at the

Battle of Wood Lake on September 23. The Dakota surrendered at Camp Release on September 28, freeing 269 captives, including 107 white settlers and 162 "mixed-bloods." An estimated 700 to 1,500 white settlers plus soldiers had been killed. Dakota casualties are not known.

A total of 392 Natives were hastily tried in September through November, and 303 were sentenced to be executed. Henry Whipple, the Episcopal bishop of Minnesota, pleaded to President Lincoln to commute the sentences of the Native warriors. Lincoln reviewed the trial records carefully and commuted the sentences of all but 38. In Lincoln's words:

> *Anxious to not act with so much clemency as to encourage another outbreak on the one hand, nor with so much severity as to be real cruelty on the other, I caused a careful examination of the records of trials to be made, in view of first ordering the execution of such as had been proved guilty of violating females. Contrary to my expectations, only two of this class were found. I then directed a further examination, and a classification of all who were proven to have participated in massacres, as distinguished from participation in battles. This class numbered forty, and included the two convicted of female violation. One of the number is strongly recommended by the commission which tried them for commutation to ten years' imprisonment. I have ordered the other thirty-nine to be executed on Friday, the 19th instant.*[18]

One additional prisoner was subsequently exonerated, leaving a final total of thirty-eight condemned. They were executed in Mankato on December 26, 1862, in the largest mass execution in U.S. history. Those whose sentences were commuted were imprisoned for four years at Camp McClellan in Davenport, Iowa, where a third died of disease and starvation. The remainder were exiled to a reservation in Nebraska.

Among the thirty-eight executed, Marpiya Okinajin, or "He Who Stands in the Clouds," was known to English speakers as "Cut-Nose." During the hostilities, he and other Natives captured a group of fleeing white settlers near Fort Ridgely. A Sisseton woman who was married to a white Indian agent interceded, and they did not harm the group.[19] Helen Clapesattle, in *The Doctors Mayo*, described him in language typical of 1941: "A fiend incarnate during the outbreak, the ringleader in all the most brutal outrages."[20] His body was buried with the others in a shallow mass grave by the river. The bodies were dug up by grave robbers and used for anatomic specimens. Dr. William Worrall Mayo lived near Le

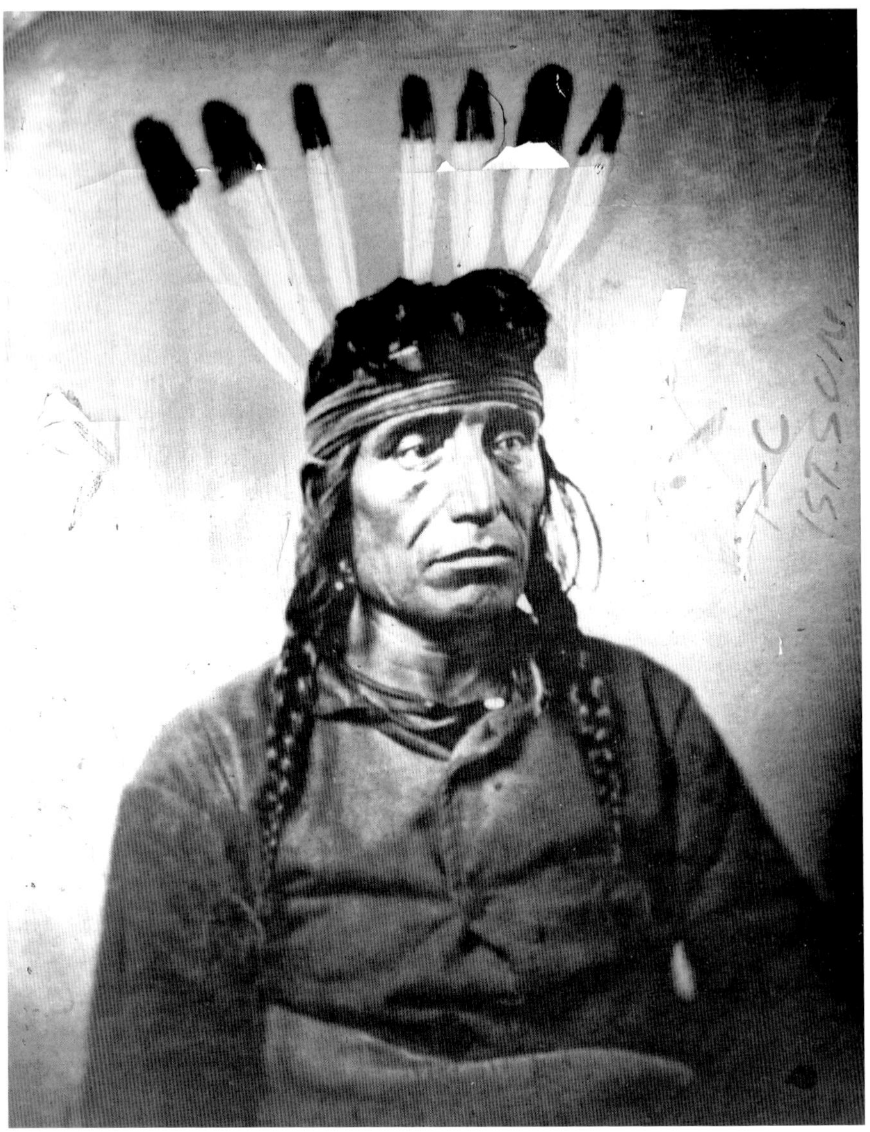

Marpiya Okinajin, known as "Cut-Nose."

Sueur at the time and participated in battle for New Ulm. He acquired the body of Marpiya Okinajin and used it for dissection and then preserved the skeleton. The Mayo brothers grew up with the skeleton in their home. From it they learned human skeletal anatomy. The passage of the Native American Graves Protection and Repatriation Act of 1990 mandated the return of Native American cultural items to descendants and affiliated tribes. Representatives of the Shakopee Mdewakanton Tribe requested the return of the remains of Marpiya Okinajin. Mayo Clinic had no record to identify his remains. In collaboration with the University of Minnesota Department of Anthropology, using a computer algorithm and a single frontal portrait photograph, they were able to identify, with a high degree of certainty, the correct skull from a number of other anatomical specimens. It was returned to the tribe and accorded appropriate burial rites in July 2000.

Taoyatiduta, which means "his people are red," was known as Little Crow. He was a fourth-generation chief of the Mdewakanton Dakota people. He (or his father, whose name was the same) had negotiated the Treaty of Mendota in 1851 and later pleaded unsuccessfully with President Buchanan for fair treatment when the government failed to honor the terms of the treaty. When members of his tribe advocated war against the white settlers, he predicted a bad outcome but reluctantly agreed to lead his people into battle. He led the attack at Fort Ridgely but probably not the attack on New Ulm. Little Crow was not captured during the hostilities but was injured and escaped to Canada. He returned to the area in July 1863, but in an altercation near Hutchinson with Nathan Lamson and his son Chauncey, he was killed, scalped and dismembered. The state legislature awarded Lamson a bounty of $500, an enormous sum at that time, for killing Little Crow. Parts of Little Crow's body were exhibited at the Minnesota Historical Society until the early twentieth century, when they were returned to his people.

After the conclusion of local hostilities, 1,600 Native women, children and old men were rounded up and kept in a prison camp on Pike Island below Fort Snelling through the harsh winter of 1862–63. Over 300 died of starvation and disease. In April, Congress declared all treaties with the Dakota null and void; the survivors were exiled to reservations in South Dakota and Nebraska, and a twenty-five-dollar-per-scalp bounty was established for any Dakota found free in Minnesota. Military actions continued against the Dakota and Lakota tribes farther west, ending with the Massacre at Wounded Knee in South Dakota in 1890. Minnesota census data from 1860 and 1870 show a drop in the Indian population from 2,369 to 690, a 71 percent decrease. None lived in Olmsted or the surrounding counties in either year.[21]

Two small groups of Dakota from different tribes that had not participated in the war remained on small reservations near Mankato. Ojibwe remained on reservations in northern Minnesota. Otherwise, until recent decades, Native Americans were unwelcomed throughout the region. Poverty, racism and stereotypes persist. Preservation of Native languages and customs is now an active process. The Native American population has increased slightly. In 2020, the population of Rochester is estimated at 115,733, including about 550 Native Americans (0.5 percent). That includes not only Dakota and Ojibwe but also members of many other nations and tribes.

A young hero of the Dakota War was eleven-year-old Merton Eastlick, whose father and three brothers were massacred. He followed the evacuation route, carrying his fifteen-month-old brother Johnny for fifty miles, saving both of their lives. Their mother was shot multiple times and left for dead but survived and was eventually reunited with her two surviving children. They were evacuated to Rochester. Mrs. Eastlick eventually moved to Mankato, but Merton settled in Rochester.[22]

Lions and Tigers and Bears, Oh My!

People sometimes speculate about apex predators in this area before white settlers. Many assume that the name of Bear Creek indicates the presence of bears in the region. In fact, it was named after Benjamin Bear, who was the first settler in Eyota in 1853. His homestead farm includes the spring from which Bear Creek arises. Bear have been rarely reported in the region. Like moose, male black bears sometimes rove out of their native northern lands during the mating season and will rarely venture into southeast Minnesota.[23]

Eaton reports that in the early days of settlement "wolves abounded, and their weird howls were nightly heard."[24] In Mitchell's 1866 *History of Olmsted County*, he reports, "This summer (1855), the wolves were quite troublesome, and committed frequent depredations on the property of persons who had neglected to put their effects out of their reach. In one instance they entered the dwelling house of Mr. Geo. Head and carried off a sheep that had been killed to furnish mutton for the breakfast of a company of travelers, though a number of persons were sleeping in the room over the one where the robbery took place."[25]

Clapesattle reported a close call that Dr. Will Mayo had when making a house call early in his career. On a snowy evening, he took a shortcut through the woods and was pursued by two wolves, which he kept at bay by "flourishing his medicine bag at the beasts to scare them off, but they followed him to the very door of his patient's cottage."[26] Coyotes and foxes, both grey and red, are common still.

Cougars (or mountain lions) included Olmsted County in their historic range but were not seen in the area for many years, until recently. They are expanding their ranges in recent years, and several sightings have been reported in Dodge County recently. Bobcats are not common but are occasionally seen in Olmsted County.

Nearly the entire weasel family can be seen in Olmsted County, including weasel, mink, otter and badger (no wolverines or fishers; pine marten are out of range here, but I was fairly confident I saw one by the Zumbro River at Seventy-Fifth Street Northwest a few years back).

Our avian predators include the biggest (golden and bald eagles) and the fastest (peregrine falcons) and a large range of hawks and owls. The National Eagle Center in Wabasha and the International Owl Center in Houston are wonderful nearby educational resources.

Of the larger herbivores, Leonard notes that "there is no reason to believe that the buffalo roamed over the Olmsted prairies; the bones or horns of the awkward beasts were not found by the first settlers, but elk were frequently seen and shot and their horns were often found. The last elk was shot on the Bamber farm by Asahel Smith, of Rochester, in 1859."[27]

The Passenger Pigeon

Leonard described the local actions that contributed to the extinction of the passenger pigeon:

> *For years the woods from Kalmar and New Haven to Pine Island were the resort, in the early summer, of wild* [passenger] *pigeons which nested there. Every morning and afternoon, during the breeding season, flocks of the birds could be seen for miles around, leaving and returning to their nests, and the Genoa woods were raided ruthlessly by hunters from the surrounding country. The pot-hunters shipped the birds and their squabs in bags and barrels to Chicago and other markets, and the breaking up of their nests and the thinning of the timber for fuel destroyed the homes of the birds, and the pigeon roosts are no more.*[28]

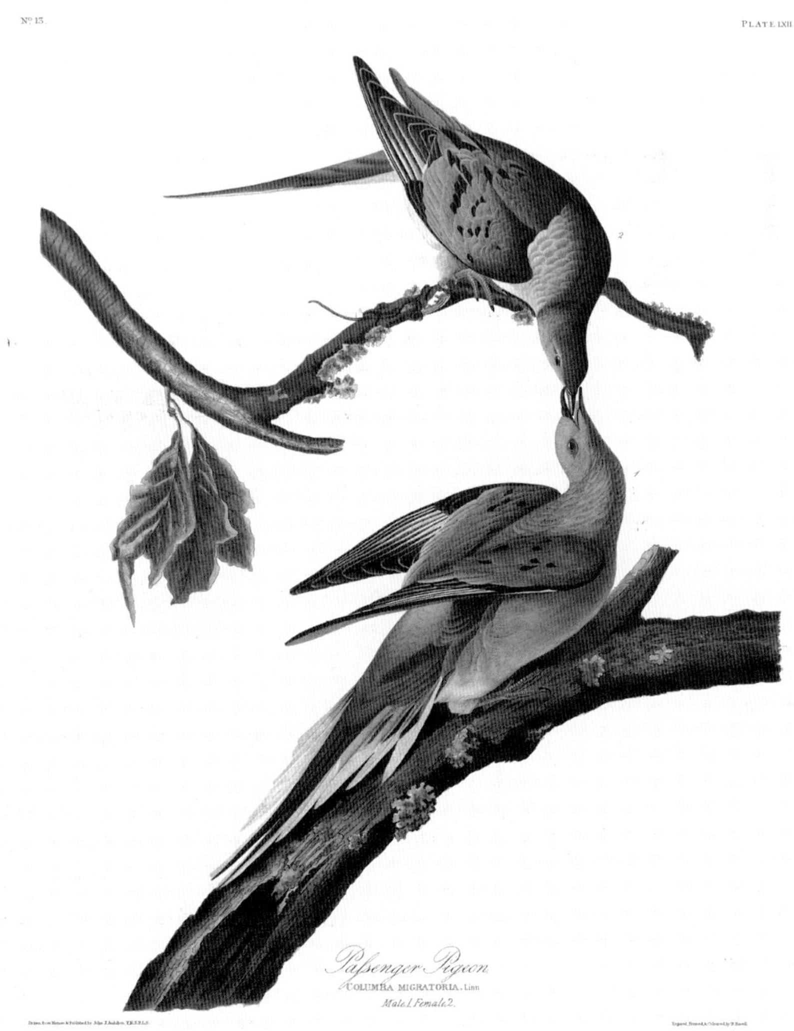

Passenger pigeon, by John James Audubon. *Courtesy of National Audubon Society.*

Passenger pigeons were once the most populous birds in North America. They flocked by the billions. They were hunted to extinction. The last wild passenger pigeon was killed by a hunter in Indiana on April 3, 1902. The last one in captivity died on September 1, 1914.

Stagecoaches to Trains to Planes

Local commerce and Mayo Clinic have depended on efficient transportation to Rochester throughout their respective histories. The earliest settlers arrived in "prairie schooners" pulled by oxen. The first stagecoach route through Rochester was established by M.O. Walker on July 15, 1854, just three days after George Head arrived in Rochester. The Dubuque Trail stretched 272 miles from Dubuque, Iowa, via Chatfield, Pleasant Grove, Rochester and Oronoco to St. Paul on a path very close to the modern U.S. Highway 52. Third Avenue Southeast was part of the route and was called Dubuque Street (memorialized by a historic plaque at 717 Third Avenue Southeast), while Seventh Street Northwest was called Oronoco Road. A remnant of the Dubuque Trail, a bridge abutment, remains in Root River County Park, the oldest man-made structure in the county. An east–west stage line was established between Winona and Mankato and stopped at Dover and Eyota to the east and Kalmar, Mantorville, Wasioja and Owatonna to the west.

On October 1, 1864, the Winona & St. Peter Railroad stopped in Rochester for the first time. It connected Winona to Rochester, allowing passenger travel between Chicago and Rochester and on to Mankato and points west. The first station was located at Civic Center Drive and First Avenue Northwest. The train's westbound line was south of the stagecoach line, dooming Kalmar (which no longer exists) in favor of Byron and favoring Kasson over Mantorville and Dodge Center over Wasioja. Passenger service lasted almost a century, until the last passenger train pulled out of Rochester on July 29, 1963. At its best, rail transport was served by the Northwestern *Rochester 400*, so named because it could travel the four-hundred-mile route in four hundred minutes. It was a daily "cannonball" from Chicago direct to Rochester. East–west traffic was carried on the Chicago and Northwestern Line while north–south traffic was carried on the Chicago and Great Western Line beginning in 1902. The C&GW depot was originally located at Fourth Street on the east riverbank, where the rail spur remains. The building that now houses Porch and Cellar Restaurants is the C&GW depot building, rebuilt two blocks to the north after the railyard fire of June 1, 1910. The *Red Bird* was the luxury express train from Rochester to St. Paul in the 1920s and '30s. It had a vermillion red coal-burning steam locomotive capable of running at up to sixty miles per hour. The train was considered the ultimate in luxury, "affording all the comforts of a well-appointed club."[29]

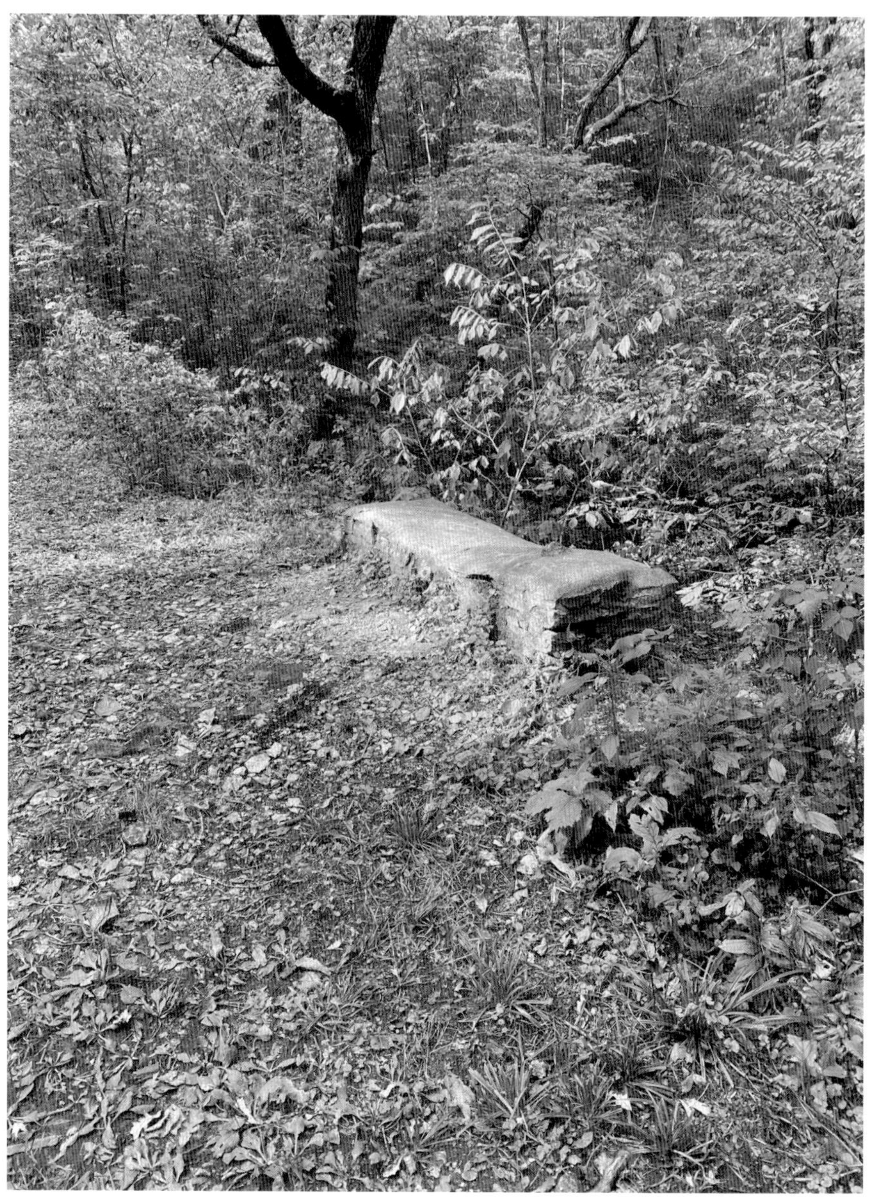

Bridge abutment from Dubuque Trail. *Courtesy of Jacob Brettin.*

NORTH WESTERN
400
ROCHESTER

The *Rochester 400*.

CHICAGO GREAT WESTERN
"RED BIRD"
NON STOP TRAIN BETWEEN
ROCHESTER—ST. PAUL—MINNEAPOLIS
All Steel Equipment
Parlor—Observation Car and Coaches
Faster than any other Way
916
CHICAGO GREAT WESTERN

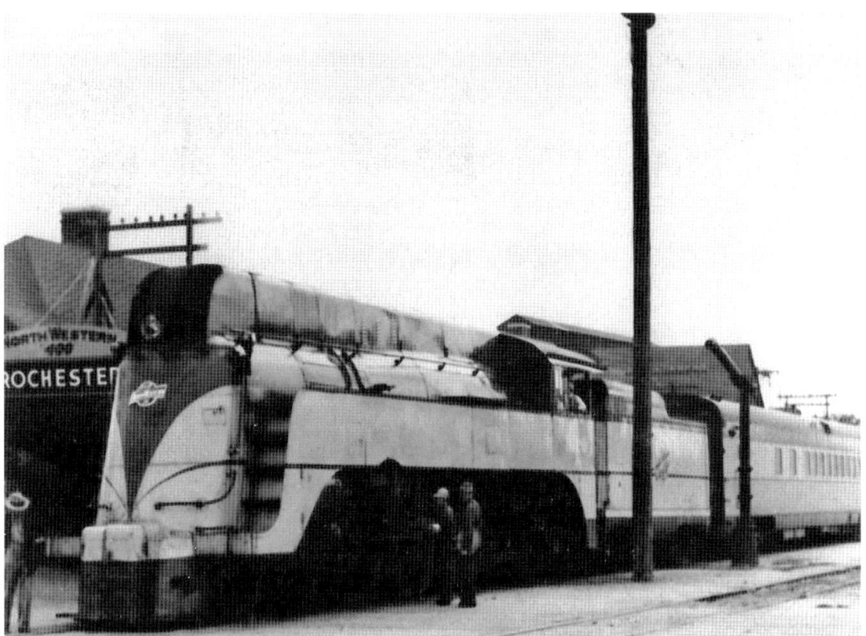

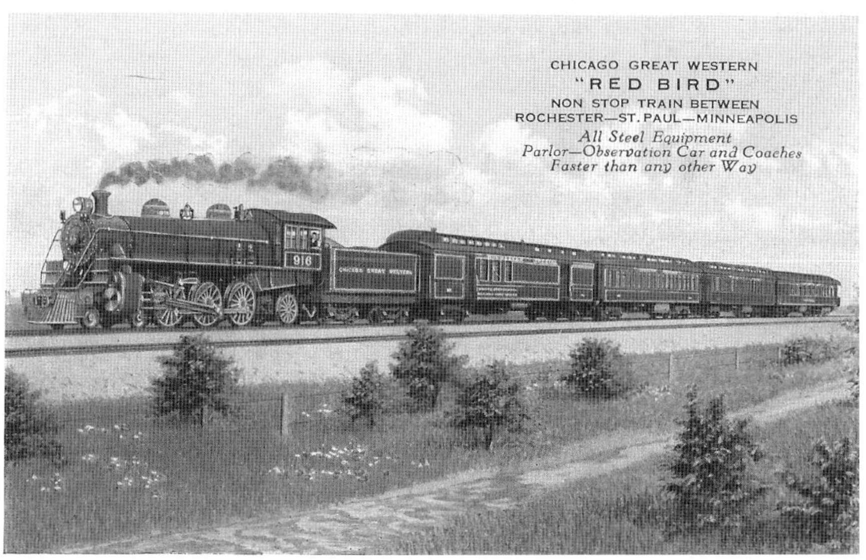

Postcard of the *Red Bird*.

Automotive traffic began in about 1900. Dr. Charlie Mayo owned the first automobile in town. Rochester is at the intersection of U.S. Highways 14, 52 and 63. The interchange with U.S. Interstate Highway 90 is nine miles south of downtown.

The first airport, called Stankey's Field, was just west of the city limits, off U.S. Highway 14 (what is now Second Street Southwest and County Road 34) in 1928. The second airport, in southeast Rochester, served the city from 1929 to 1961. It was operated by Rochester Airport Company, a subsidiary of Mayo Foundation, to provide for transportation of Mayo Clinic patients. It was initially owned by Mayo Clinic, but in 1945, Mayo Clinic transferred ownership of the field to the City of Rochester. In 1952, it was named after Albert J. Lobb, a Mayo Clinic administrator and the first airport director. Its proximity to downtown necessitated a sweeping beacon mounted on the top of the Plummer Building. Airmail service began on March 8, 1930. Lobb Field was expanded, and runways were paved in 1940. After Lobb Field was decommissioned, the vacated runways and fields were used to build the Meadow Park neighborhood, Ben Franklin Elementary School and Mayo High School.

The current Rochester International Airport, seven and a half miles southwest of downtown, began service on August 19, 1961, and expanded in 1975. It has multiple daily flights to Minneapolis/St. Paul International

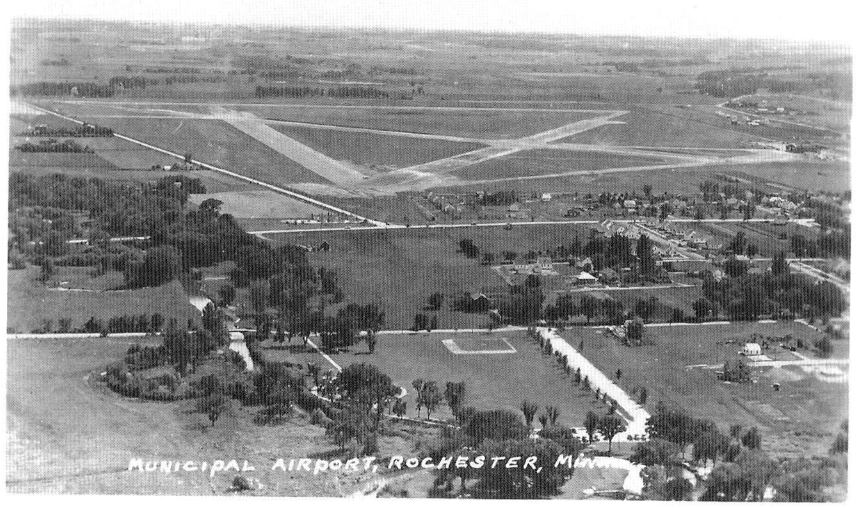

Aerial postcard of Lobb Field from northeast over Bear Creek.

Airport on Delta Air Lines, to Chicago's O'Hare Airport on American and United Airlines and to Denver International Airport on United Airlines. It achieved international status in 1995. It is still operated by Mayo Clinic. It has six gates in a commercial terminal, plus a separate general aviation terminal that supports private, charter and international flights and a FedEx Express terminal. The commercial terminal is named in honor of Mark G. "Jerry" Brataas, longtime Mayo Clinic administrator and promoter of air transportation.

Dee Cabin

The oldest wooden structure in Rochester is a log cabin. It was built with poplar logs in the spring of 1862 by William Dee. It has two rooms and a loft. It was originally located at what is now 428 Sixth Street Southwest. The Dees lived in the cabin for four years with their four children. Subsequent owners were Mr. A.D. Robinson, Mr. Ole Swenson and his daughter, Mrs. Frank Graham and finally Mr. Andrew Seeverts.[30] In July 1911, Mr. Seeverts donated the forty-nine-year-old cabin to Mayo Park in honor of his friend Dr. William Worrall Mayo. It was kept for many years on the east side of

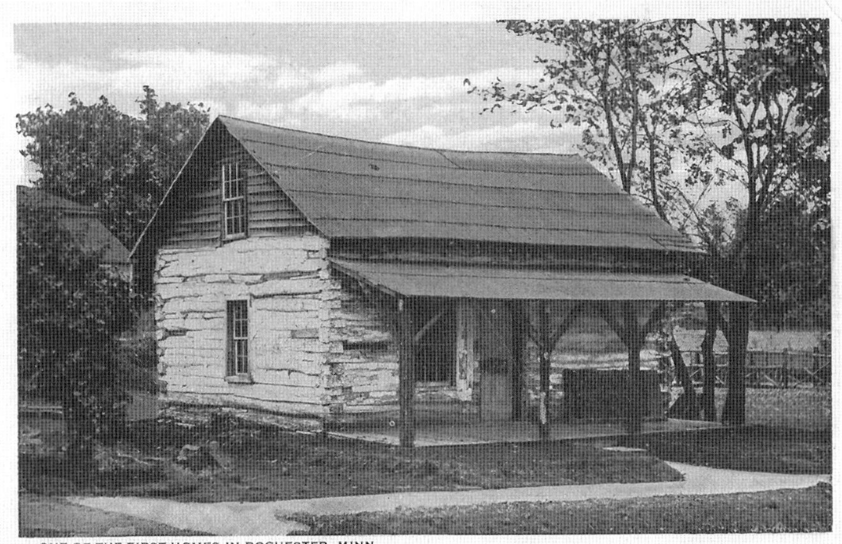

Postcard of Dee Cabin.

the river on high ground, featured as part of a small zoo. In 1962, the cabin was moved from Mayo Park to a site next to the History Center of Olmsted County at 214 Third Avenue Southwest. In 1974, the History Center of Olmsted County was built on West Circle Drive by Salem Road Southwest, and the cabin was moved to the grounds of the History Center.

Civil War—An Oxymoron

Recruitment for the war began after the attack on Fort Sumter on April 12, 1861. Governor Ramsey happened to be in Washington and was the first official to pledge troops—one thousand from the First Minnesota Regiment. That group was recruited primarily from St. Paul and the surrounding area. The first large group from the Rochester area was Company B of the Second Minnesota Regiment, under the command of Captain William Markham (later Colonel Markham). Colonel James George said, "The Second never misunderstood an order, never charged the rebels without driving them, was never charged by the rebels but the rebels were repulsed and never retreated under fire of the enemy." They were noted particularly for their distinguished service in the battles of Mill Springs and Chickamauga.

Olmsted residents also contributed substantially to Companies C and K of the Third Regiment, Company I of the Fifth Regiment, Company H of the Sixth Regiment, Company D of the Eighth Regiment, Company F of the Ninth Regiment and Company H of the Eleventh Regiment Minnesota Infantry, as well as Company H of the First Regiment Heavy Artillery, Company I of the First Regiment Mounted Rangers, Company L of the Second Regiment Minnesota Cavalry, Companies C and D of Brackett's Battalion of the Minnesota Cavalry and Companies F, G, H and I of the First Battalion. In the disastrous Battle of Guntown, 23 Olmsted residents of the Ninth Regiment were captured and suffered terribly or died at the hands of the enemy, many at the infamous Andersonville Prison. Company K of the Third Regiment was badly outnumbered (700 infantry versus 2,800 cavalry) at the Battle of Murfreesboro and was forced to surrender. They were spared the horrors of Confederate prisons by a prisoner exchange. They subsequently regrouped in Minnesota in September 1862 and acquitted their reputation by effective and nearly bloodless performance in the Dakota War and subsequent assignments farther south, until they were mustered out of service in September 1865.

A total of 2,128,948 soldiers served in the Union army, including about 22,000 from Minnesota, of whom about 2,500 died. Out of a population of 12,000, Olmsted County contributed 1,333 participants (275 from Rochester), 1,191 volunteers and 142 conscripts.[31]

W.W. Mayo Comes to Town, 1863

William Worrall Mayo is the subject of the first 207 pages of Helen Clapesattle's *The Doctors Mayo*, as well as Judith Hartzell's *I Started This: The Life of Dr. William Worrall Mayo.* Although his achievements are sometimes overshadowed by his famous sons, he was a pioneer physician, a very skilled surgeon, the third president of the Minnesota Medical Association, a great mentor and a great advocate for education, the role of women in medicine and care of the oppressed or downtrodden.

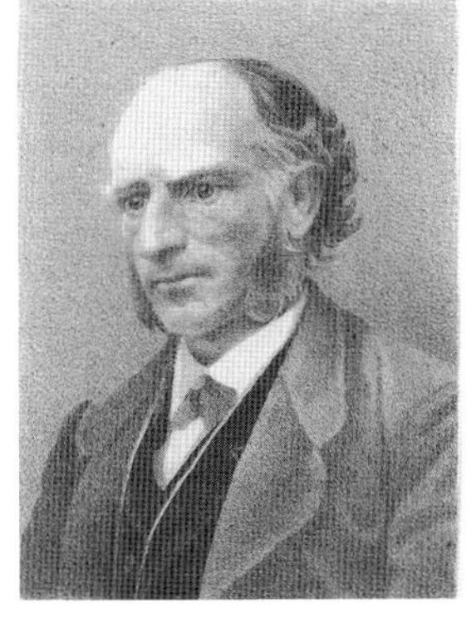

William Worrall Mayo, mid-career. *From Andreas's* Historical Atlas of the State of Minnesota, *1874.*

W.W. Mayo was born near Salford, in Lancashire, England, on May 31, 1819. He claimed to have been a pupil of the famous chemist John Dalton at the University of Manchester. He immigrated to the United States in 1846, at the age of twenty-seven. He worked briefly as a pharmacist at Bellevue Hospital in New York. He moved west to Lafayette, Indiana, where he studied medicine at Indiana Medical College and apprenticed with Dr. Elizur Deming. He married Louise Wright in 1851. Their first child, Gertrude, was born in Lafayette.

Dr. Mayo received a second medical degree from the University of Missouri. Finances were tight, and Louise established a successful millinery business (women's hats). While in Indiana, Mayo was stricken by a recurrent febrile illness resembling malaria. Louise recounted years later that in the summer of 1854, "one morning…in the midst of an attack of chills and fever, he hitched up his rig and said to me, 'Good-bye, Louise. I am going to keep on driving until I get well or die.'"[32] He left Indiana and traveled to the Minnesota Territory in 1854. He encouraged Louise to move to St. Paul, where she reestablished her business very successfully. Because there was a plethora of physicians, Dr. Mayo made his living in St. Paul as a tailor.

Indulging his wanderlust further, he made multiple trips through wilderness to St. Louis County (subsequent site of Duluth, Minnesota), where he made a land claim and practiced medicine. He chaired the first St. Louis County board of commissioners. In 1859, he and Louise moved near Le Sueur on the Minnesota River in "Sioux Country," newly open to white settlers. They were active participants in the Dakota War, described earlier. Their son William James was born in Le Sueur.

On April 24, 1863, Mayo was appointed by President Lincoln as examining surgeon for draftees to the Union army in the Southern District of Minnesota, headquartered in Rochester. He served until February 1865, when he was accused of impropriety in his examinations. He was ultimately exonerated. After leaving that position, he wanted to return to practice in St. Paul, but Louise refused to move from Rochester. He established his home and practice in Rochester, but in May 1873, he was persuaded to join a practice in St. Paul. Louise and the children stayed in Rochester, and he commuted back to Rochester to visit. The following March, he was marooned in Kasson by a blizzard that stopped train travel for several days. Too impatient to wait, he walked home eighteen miles through untracked snow. He survived the trip but decided to abandon his St. Paul practice and returned to Rochester. (See "Blizzards" on page 175.)

The senior Dr. Mayo was a respected general practitioner in the Rochester area. He was a talented and innovative surgeon in the period before aseptic technique. Known as the "Little Doctor" or the "Old Doctor," he dressed meticulously in a top hat and coat tails on house calls. He was also a notoriously hurried carriage driver and frequently passed slower carriages in his way. He was well respected in the Minnesota Medical Association and served as its third president. He was active in local politics and served two terms as a pugnacious Democrat mayor of Rochester, as well as several terms on the school board. He led the medical team that cared for the injured after the tornado in 1883, and he agreed to be the medical director of St. Marys Hospital when it opened in 1889. He retired from active practice and surgery in 1892, at age seventy-three, but continued to see patients in consultation. He served in the Minnesota State Senate from 1891 to 1895. Late in life, he traveled extensively. According to Mayo family lore, he was ejected from a bullfight in Mexico City for cheering for the bull.[33] In 1907, he took a two-month excursion to Japan and China, sponsored by railroad baron James J. Hill. They were friends from riverboat days when the Mayos lived in Le Sueur. He celebrated his eighty-eighth birthday aboard Hill's steamship *Minnesota* on the return trip across the Pacific.[34]

His mentorship of his sons is accepted as a given, though they always emphasized his and Louise's importance in their careers. Often forgotten is his critical mentorships of pharmaceutical magnate and philanthropist Sir Henry Wellcome and attorney Frank B. Kellogg, who became a trust buster, senator, ambassador, secretary of state and Nobel peace laureate. Little is recorded of his relationship with James J. Hill or why Hill was so extravagant with Mayo late in life.

He died on March 6, 1911, at the age of ninety-one of complications from a crush injury to his hand and forearm. Sister Joseph Dempsey said of him: "He was an alert, able, earnest humanitarian, worthy of all the glory his sons have added to his name." He is buried at Oakwood Cemetery beside his wife, Louise, his daughter Phoebe and his two famous sons. The larger-than-life bronze statue of W.W. Mayo by Leonard Crunelle of Chicago was commissioned by the citizens of Rochester after his death. It stood for many years in the Statuary Park (north of Second Street, east of First Avenue Southeast), then at the west end of the Mayo Memorial Mall. It now stands with a similarly scaled contemporary bronze of Mother Alfred Moes by Mike Major in the Feith Family Statuary Park west of the Gonda Entrance.

Old Central School, 1868

Public school facilities in early Rochester were primitive for the first twelve years. The first school, built in the spring of 1856, was a log structure at what is now Fifth Street between Second and Third Avenues Southeast (in the Fullerton parking lot). It served as a church and election polling place as well as a school. Mary Walker was the first teacher. Subsequently, school was taught in a variety of buildings, often as a secondary use of crude log public buildings. Over one hundred schools, mostly small and rural, were established in Olmsted County by 1866. That year, Rochester voted to improve its educational facilities. With almost no opposition, a levy was approved by popular vote to build two small brick schools in the first (Hawthorne School) and third (Phelps, later Edison) wards plus Central School on Zumbro (Second) Street, where the Mayo Building is now.

Two years later, a magnificent brick and stone five-story facility was dedicated with sixteen classrooms and twin towers that made it the tallest building in Minnesota. It was 94 by 87 feet; the taller of its two towers was 127 feet. The north tower was 100 feet tall and held a 1,551-pound

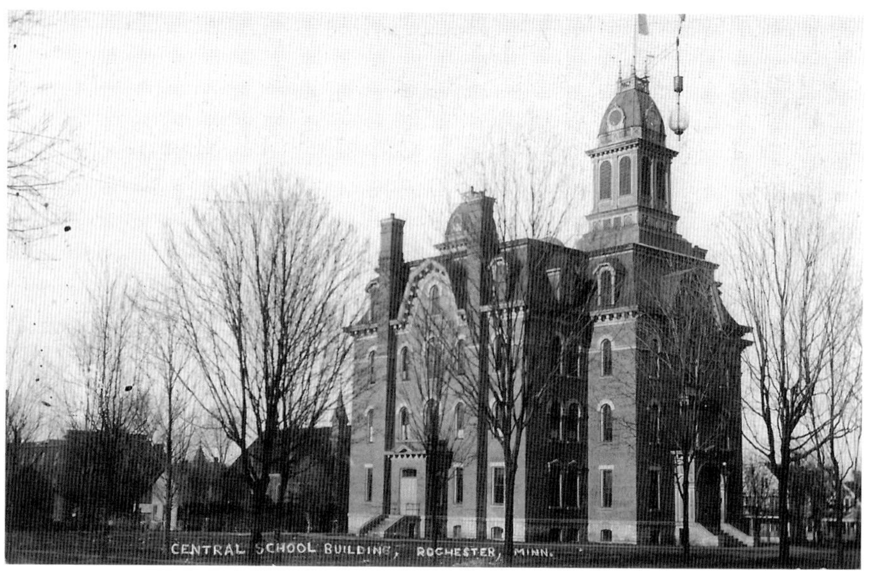

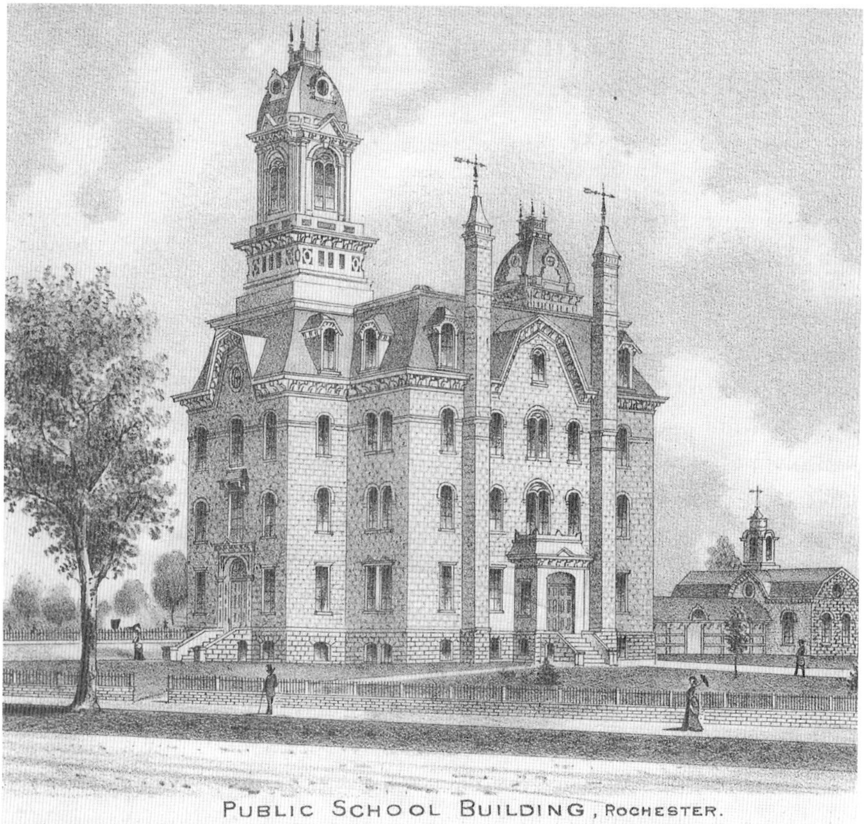

PUBLIC SCHOOL BUILDING, ROCHESTER.

E.W. CROSS, M.D. President Board of Education. C.S. YOUNGLOVE, Clerk.

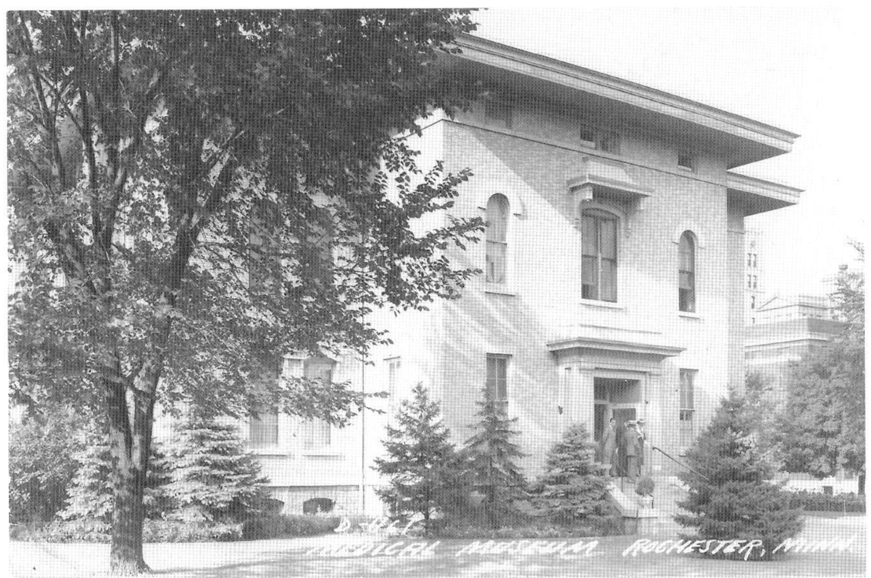

Opposite, top: Postcard of Old Central School.

Opposite, bottom: Central School. *From Andreas's* Historical Atlas of the State of Minnesota, *1874*.

Above: Postcard of Central School, which after a fire and new roof became Mayo Medical Museum.

bell[35] used thereafter to toll the quarter hours. It also served as the town fire alarm, heard throughout the city. W.W. Mayo was a member of the school board that approved and built Central, and the Mayo brothers attended and became alumni of the school.

Central served the community well until September 1, 1910, when a fire destroyed the top two floors and the towers. A new high school was built two blocks to the west, and the Central School remains were salvaged by building a new low pitch roof over the remaining three floors. It functioned as a school until it was acquired by Mayo Clinic in the 1920s, after which it housed the Mayo Medical Museum on the first floor and provided expansion office space on the upper levels. It was torn down in 1950 to make way for the Mayo Building. The medical museum was then housed in a Quonset hut and after 1963 in the Damon Parkade. Despite numerous requests over the years, the medical museum has not been reestablished since it was removed from the Damon Parkade. Mayo Clinic historical archives and artifacts are maintained by the W. Bruce Fye Center for the History of Medicine on the third floor of the Plummer Building.

Henry S. Wellcome

Henry Solomon Wellcome was born on August 21, 1853, in a prairie log cabin in Almond, Wisconsin, the son of an itinerant preacher. Early in childhood, his family moved to Garden City, Minnesota, near Mankato. His ninth birthday occurred during the Dakota War. He was deeply impressed by the plight of the homeless refugees, as well as injustices to the Natives. When he was thirteen, his father joined his physician uncle in running a pharmacy in Garden City. Henry worked as an assistant. At age seventeen, he moved to Rochester and took a job as a pharmacy clerk at the Geisinger and Newton Drug Store. W.W. Mayo saw promise in the young man and instructed him in chemistry and physics and loaned him books. He encouraged him to seek further education and supported him financially to attend first the Chicago College of Pharmacy (destroyed by the Great Chicago Fire on October 10, 1871) and then the Philadelphia College of Pharmacy, from which he graduated in 1874.

He worked two years in sales for Caswell Hazard & Co., a large New York pharmaceutical firm, and then with McKesson and Robbins. In 1880, with encouragement from the Mayos,[36] he partnered with Silas Mainville Burroughs to create Burroughs and Wellcome, incorporated in London. They introduced medicines in tablet form, a much more convenient and portable form than liquid or powdered medications, in Great Britain and subsequently the British Empire. They developed innovative marketing and very quickly became one of the largest pharmaceutical manufacturers in the world. Burroughs died in 1895 at age forty-eight, leaving Wellcome (aged forty-two) as the sole owner of the company. In 1903, he established the Wellcome Tropical Research Laboratories in Khartoum, Sudan, for study of tropical diseases. Then in 1913, he created the Wellcome Bureau for Scientific Research. He supported research to develop antitoxins for tetanus, diphtheria and gas gangrene, as well as the isolation of histamine, leading to production of antihistamines, and the standardization of insulin and

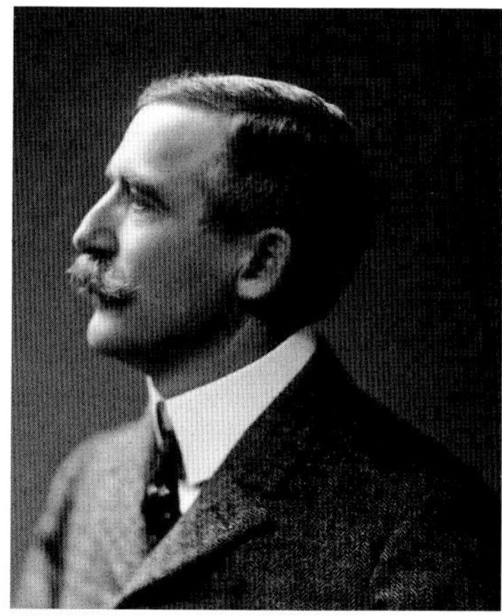

Henry S. Wellcome sends regards to Dr. Charlie Mayo. *By permission of Mayo Foundation for Medical Education and Research.*

other medications. He became a British subject in 1910 and was knighted in 1932. The same year, he became an honorary fellow of the Royal College of Surgeons of England.

He acquired enormous wealth and an extensive collection of medical and archaeological artifacts. In 1913, he founded the Wellcome Historical Medical Museum to exhibit them. Some have subsequently been displayed at the Science Museum in London, some in the Wellcome Collection and some in the Wellcome Library. He also expended considerable money and effort in defense of the rights of Native Americans.

In his will, Wellcome left his estate to the Wellcome Trust. The trustees were charged to spend the income for human and animal health and to foster the study of medical history through the maintenance and exhibition of his collections. In 1986 and 1995, the Wellcome Trust sold its interest in the Wellcome Foundation, which thus became part of Glaxo Wellcome and eventually GlaxoSmithKline or GSK, the world's largest pharmaceutical company. The trust's endowment is currently valued at $40.2 billion, making it the fourth-largest charitable foundation in the world (after Novo Nordisk, $73.1 billion; Stichting INGKA, $61.8 billion; and Bill and Melinda Gates, $49.9). It provides over $600 million per year in research and educational funding. Priorities include biomedical science, technology transfer and bioethics. The Wellcome Trust is the largest private funder of medical research in Britain. Its influence is so great that seventeen Wellcome-funded scientists have become fellows of the Royal Society. Sir Henry Dale received the 1936 Nobel Prize in Physiology or Medicine for his work with acetylcholine. Gertrude Elion and George Hitchings won the 1988 Nobel Prize in Physiology or Medicine for work with antiviral agents done at Wellcome Research Laboratories. The research directors of many British pharmaceutical companies were trained under Wellcome-funded programs.

The Burroughs Wellcome Fund (BWF) is a separate United States–based entity, created in 1955. Since receiving a $400 million gift from the Wellcome Trust in 1993, the BWF has been an independent private medical research foundation based in Research Triangle Park, North Carolina. In 2017, BWF was valued at just under $770 million.

Wellcome maintained his friendship with and admiration for W.W. Mayo and was a friend and correspondent of both Mayo brothers. He visited Rochester throughout his life, both as a patient and as a guest of the Mayos.[37] He died of pneumonia at age eighty-two in 1936. His secretary notified the Mayos by telegram.[38] He visited Rochester the year before his death. The *Post Bulletin* quoted him as saying, "I owe whatever success I have attained in the world to Dr. William Worrall Mayo, the father of Dr. William J. and Charles H. Mayo, who took an interest in me and gave me my start."[39]

ANDREAS'S *HISTORICAL ATLAS OF THE STATE OF MINNESOTA*, 1874

A.T. Andreas's *An Illustrated Historical Atlas of the State of Minnesota* was published in 1874 to promote immigration to the state of Minnesota, established in 1858. It included plat maps of all of the counties; maps of most cities and towns; hundreds of images of businesses, churches and residences; several hundred portraits of prominent citizens, including

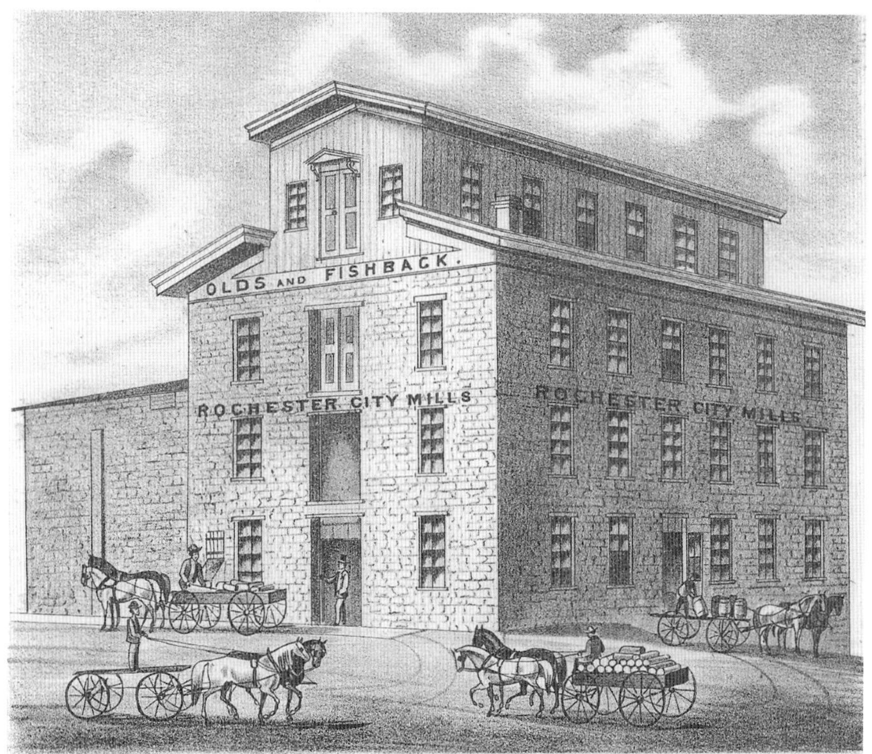

MILL OF OLDS & FISHBACK, FOOT OF 3RD ST., ROCHESTER, MINN.

OLMSTED CO. COURT HOUSE, ROCHESTER, MINNESOTA.
THOS. BROOKS, Chairman Board of Com'S

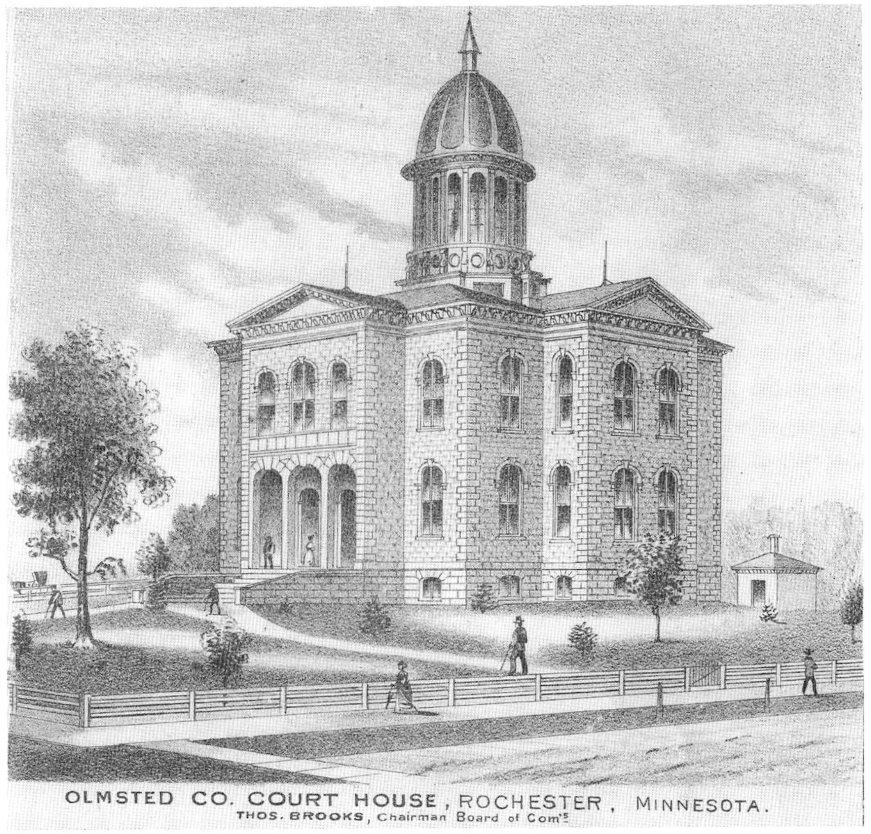

Opposite: Olds & Fishback Mill. *From Andreas's* Historical Atlas of the State of Minnesota, *1874.*

Above: Olmsted County Courthouse. *From Andreas's* Historical Atlas of the State of Minnesota, *1874.*

W.W. Mayo (almost no women); histories of the state and of each county and most towns; biographical sketches of prominent citizens; 80 pages of statistics; and a detailed list of sponsoring patrons. In addition to city and county maps, images from Rochester and Olmsted County include Olmsted County Courthouse, St. John's Catholic Church, Schuster Brewery, Olds & Fishback Mill, the W.W. Mayo residence, eighteen other residences and sixteen other businesses. It is a tome of 394 pages and is 15 by 17.5 inches and weighs 10 pounds. Intact copies are rare because map dealers unbind them to sell individual pages for ten to fifty dollars, depending on the images. For example, pages 115 and 116, front and back, include maps of

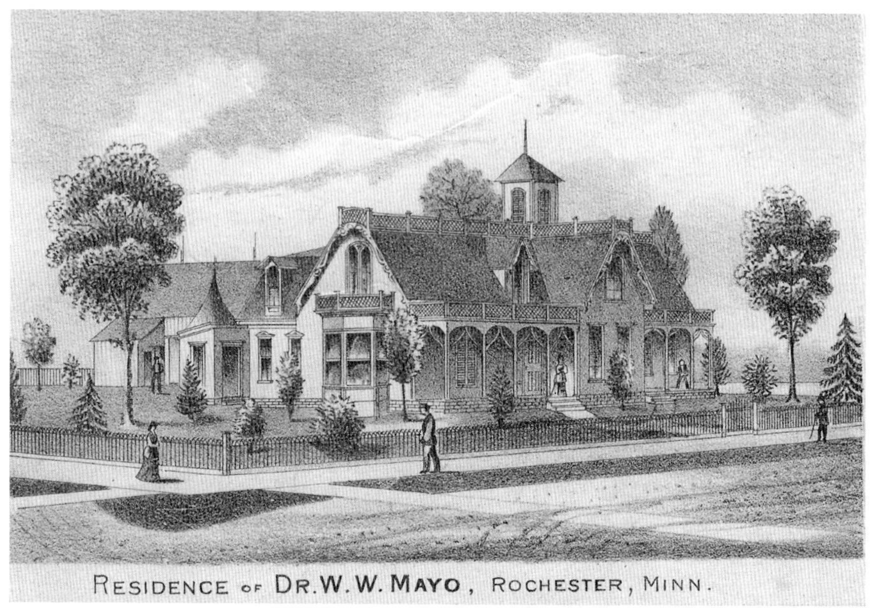

W.W. Mayo residence. *From Andreas's* Historical Atlas of the State of Minnesota, *1874.*

both Rochester and Olmsted County. The book was reprinted in smaller (11.5 by 14 inches) format without color by the Winona County Historical Society in 1976. Those copies are also rare.

Gunfight, 1877

The Honorable Joseph A. Leonard, author of the 1910 *History of Olmsted County*, was an attorney and later a judge. His history contains many reports of crimes and judicial outcomes. Minnesota was the Far West when it was established, and frontier life was rough.

Henry Kalb was a German immigrant who came to Rochester in 1856 at the age of twenty-three. He was elected city marshal in 1877 and served in that role for twenty-three years. He was described as quiet and unassuming but strict in law enforcement. On June 15, 1879, Dan Ganey committed a burglary in Owatonna. He was arrested in Kasson but escaped. Early the next morning, he ate breakfast at the Norton House, where Kalb apprehended him. Kalb accompanied him on foot to a planned meeting with a marshal from Kasson. As they crossed Broadway at what is now Center Street, Ganey broke free, pulled a revolver and told Kalb, "You go." Kalb stood his ground, and Ganey fired at close range, barely missing Kalb's cheek. Kalb returned fire but missed with his first shot. Ganey fled on foot, and Kalb pursued him. When cornered, Ganey turned and fired again but missed. Kalb then returned fire, striking Ganey in the chest and killing him.

A search of Ganey's body revealed burglary tools, a watch taken in Owatonna and a diamond shirt stud stolen from the governor's home in St. Paul, among other items. Kalb was rewarded by the citizens of Rochester with a fine gold watch and chain. He also received a gold-mounted ebony cane from Governor C.K. Davis.[40]

Second Minnesota Hospital for the Insane, 1879

In 1873, the state legislature approved a tax on alcohol to fund a Minnesota Inebriate Asylum. It was decided that it would be built in Rochester. In 1876, 160 acres of land was purchased east of town. Construction began in 1877. Political pressure caused the facility to be repurposed and renamed—before it opened—as the Second Minnesota Hospital for the Insane to ease overcrowding at St. Peter. It opened in 1879. It had a beautiful college-like campus and grounds with gardens featuring exotic plants. Treatment in the premedication era consisted of physical labor/farming, exercise and occupational therapy. For violent patients, physical restraint was sometimes used. A scandal occurred in 1889, when a Black patient named Taylor Combs, a formerly enslaved man, died. His death was initially attributed to a fall but was eventually traced to abuse by two poorly supervised attendants. On investigation, a culture of abuse, intimidation and coverup was revealed. The two attendants were found guilty of his death and were sentenced to prison. Though vindicated of wrongdoing, the hospital's first superintendent, Dr. J.E. Bowers, resigned and was replaced in 1890 by Dr. A.F. Kilbourne. He was an innovative leader and served many years in that role. Under his leadership, the hospital developed an excellent nurse training program. The first class graduated in 1892 and the last in 1968.

In 1893, the name was changed to the Rochester State Hospital. One of the mainstays of treatment was work on the hospital's 520-acre (plus 440 rented acres) farm that produced much of the food for the facility. Leonard's

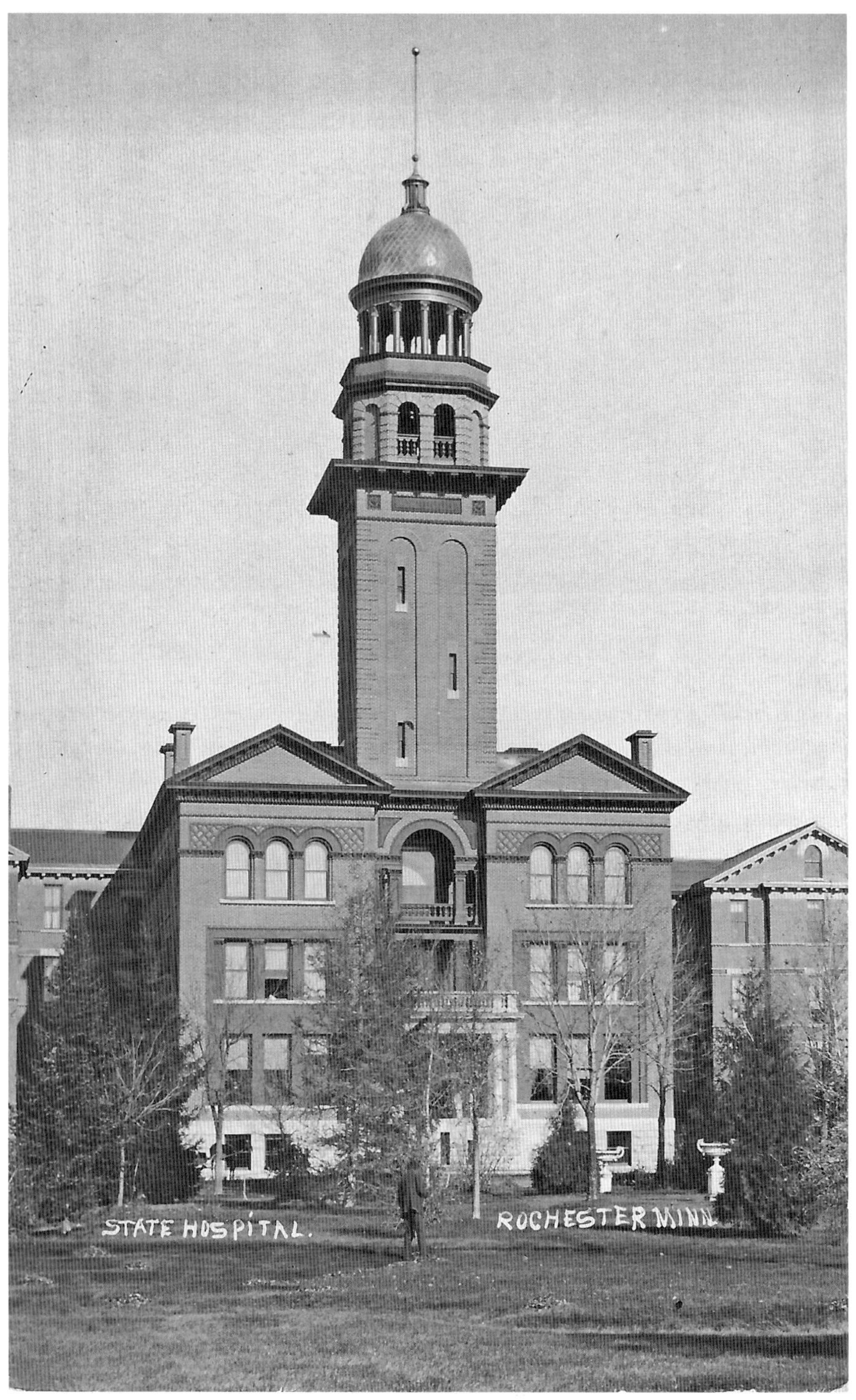
STATE HOSPITAL.
ROCHESTER MINN

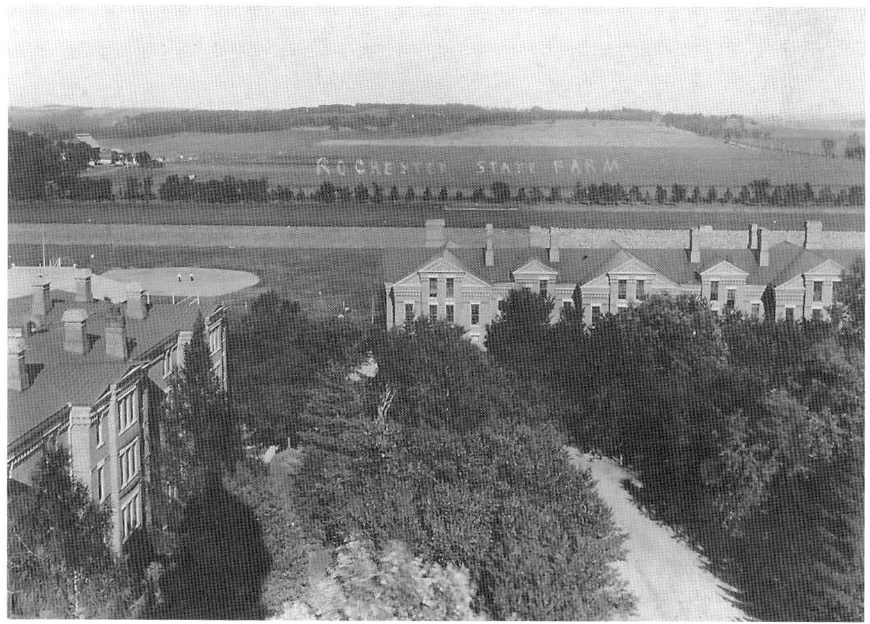

Opposite: Postcard of Rochester State Hospital Main Building.

Above: Postcard of Rochester State Hospital and grounds from tower of Main Building (note shadow).

history mentions the caves carved into the sandstone hillsides of what is now Quarry Hill Park, in which were stored thousands of bushels of produce to feed the inmates of the state hospital during the winter and spring. At that time (1908), the inpatient population was 1,161, with a total staff of 202 employees, including 116 nurses (of whom 54 percent were women).

Treatments evolved over time, but after 1940, they included insulin, electroshock therapy and lobotomy. As treatment methods changed, the old college-like campus became obsolete. Most of the original buildings were replaced between 1948 and 1964. The introduction of effective psychotropic medications in the 1960s and 1970s and a change in culture resulted in evolution toward outpatient treatment and community-based facilities.

Through most of its history, the Mayos, and subsequently Mayo Clinic, provided medical care that required specialized care, including advanced surgical procedures. It became the sole surgical referral center for the entire state hospital system, as well as the Department of Public Welfare in 1971.

In 1981, in a controversial move, the Minnesota legislature ordered Rochester State Hospital to be closed as a "cost-saving" measure, regardless

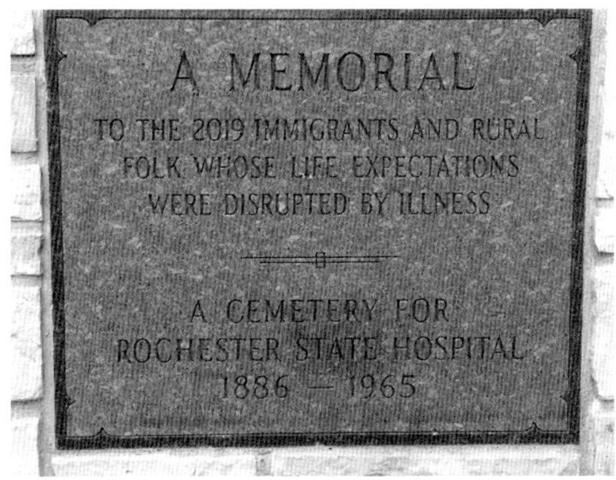

Memorial stone at Rochester State Hospital Cemetery.

of the superior care coordinated with Mayo Clinic. Despite protests, the hospital closed in June 1982.

In 1965, the state hospital sold 212 acres of its farm to the City of Rochester as part of Quarry Hill Park. This included a cemetery on a hillside with graves of 2,019 patients who died at the state hospital between 1886 and 1965. The location of a small burial plot used from 1879 to 1886 is unknown. Originally marked with wooden crosses with anonymous patient numbers, the cemetery was neglected. In 1999, efforts were begun by Roland Anderson and Berdine Erickson to place a memorial in the cemetery. After that, efforts were made to locate and mark all graves with granite gravestones. Many volunteers of the Rochester State Hospital Cemetery Recognition Group participated. Funding was provided by the Minnesota State Legislature, the City of Rochester, Olmsted County and the Carl & Verna Schmidt Foundation, with in-kind support provided by Anderson's Rochester Granite and Monument Co. The project was completed in 2016, with all graves marked.

The Federal Medical Center (FMC) of Rochester is a prison hospital for federal inmates, established in 1984, reusing some former state hospital buildings. Other buildings outside the FMC facility are used for Olmsted County Public Health Services, planning and other county offices.[41]

Geology: Karst, Caves, Sinkholes and Mounds

The old histories devote substantial space to local geology, not surprisingly, since agriculture depends heavily on geology. New settlers obtained many of their resources from local minerals, waters and other geologic resources.[42] Southern Minnesota was mostly rolling prairie, oak savannah and floodplain forests. Expanses of "Big Woods" (*Grand Bois* to French-speaking explorers) filled much of northwest Olmsted County (New Haven and Kalmar Townships). These are temperate hardwood forests of mature elm, basswood, sugar maple and red oak with hackberry, ash and aspen understory. In a state with over ten thousand lakes, Olmsted County has none and no mountains, either. In southeast Minnesota, all topography is down, not up. Valleys cut down from the plains to varying depths, some with striking bluffs, but none more than a few hundred feet in elevation.

What is Karst topography? Most of the rock in southeast Minnesota is limestone, made of either calcite ($CaCO_3$) or dolomite ($CaMg(CO_3)_2$). Limestone is soluble in acidic solutions. When water absorbs carbon dioxide from the air or from the soil, it forms carbonic acid, which is capable of dissolving limestone. As acidified water runs through cracks and crevices in limestone, it can dissolve away the stone. Groundwater is very sensitive to contamination in karst areas because of rapid transit of water through cracked limestone. When crevices reach human size, they become caves. Some are extensive. There are many in southeast Minnesota, the "mother lode of spelunking opportunities in Minnesota." Mystery Cave and Niagara Cave are the best known, but there are many more in "a vast selection of caves."[43]

There are also many sinkholes, which are formed by the same process, just below the surface. They can appear suddenly when a hole forms underground and the surface material above collapses suddenly from lack of support. This is picturesque in uninhabited woods but can be catastrophic under a house or a road. Leonard described an incident in Rochester Township in 1870 in which five horses spent a rainy night in a pasture and were discovered the following morning tumbled into a pit twelve feet wide at the top and eighteen feet deep. Fortunately, none was injured.[44] There are over eight hundred sinkholes in southeast Minnesota ranging from three to more than one hundred feet in diameter and from one to more than one hundred feet deep. They can occur virtually anywhere in Olmsted County, except several very low spots in riverbeds. They are most common southeast of Rochester in Orion, Pleasant Grove, Marion and Eyota Townships. The sites closer to Rochester with the greatest potential for sinkholes are Mayowood and east of Oronoco. The Minnesota Geological Survey map of sinkholes in Olmsted County states, "A sinkhole can form almost anywhere in Olmsted county. Although a sinkhole is more likely to form near existing sink holes,

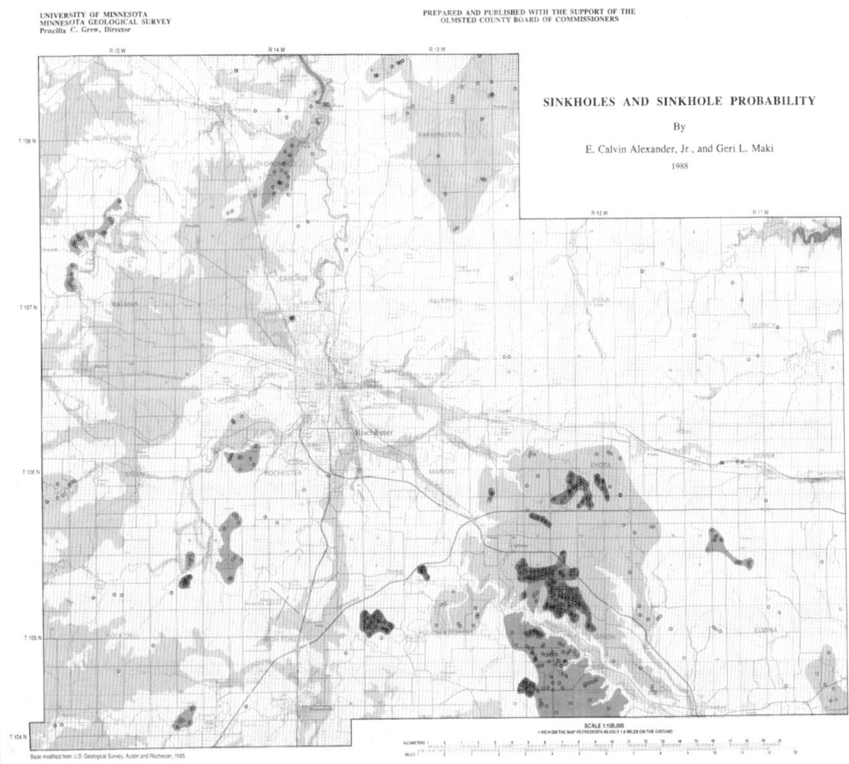

Sinkholes in Olmsted County, 1988. Details of the map are accessible through endnote reference. *Courtesy of Minnesota Geological Survey.*

Murphy's Law predicts that it will form in the least desirable place i.e. under whatever you are trying to do!"[45] The unexpected discovery of a large and very deep sinkhole under Miracle Mile added $1.3 million in remediation costs to a recent redevelopment project.[46]

There are several well-known man-made caves in Rochester. The caves in the south-facing slopes of Quarry Hill Park were part of the state hospital grounds, used for storage of produce to feed the inmates. They are carved into the St. Peter layer of sandstone. In recent years, they have been secured with locked entries for safety and for protection of the resident bats. They are opened by Quarry Hill staff on occasion for educational programs.

The caves on the south-facing slopes of the grounds of Rochester Community and Technical College are very similar in design. They were carved out of the sandstone hill in 1883 for William D. Hurlbut and James N. Coe, partners in real estate. They were intended to house hogs in a naturally cool space. The venture failed, and the caves were abandoned. Local legend has called them "Horse Thief Caves," sometimes mistakenly attributed to Jesse James and his gang, though the infamous James-Younger Gang raid in Northfield occurred in 1876, and Jesse James was killed in 1882, the year before the caves were excavated. However, there might be truth to the name. The biography *Cy Thomson, The Generous Embezzler*, describes "the locally celebrated Wells Gang [comrades of the James-Younger Gang], reputed to be horse thieves extraordinary," who stole horses throughout northern Iowa in the 1880s and '90s and shipped them to a "subterranean stable on the outskirts of Rochester," from which they were sold.[47]

Another curious local geological feature is the sandstone mounds (not Indian mounds) seen best on either side of U.S. Highway 63 north of the roundabout at Seventy-Fifth Street (County Road 14). Lone Mound is northwest of Potsdam (west of Plainview). Some are also present in eastern parts of Rochester but are obscured by excavation and development. The isolated hill west of Broadway at Northern Heights Drive and the hill behind ShopKO North have the same structure. Such mounds can be as tall as 150 feet.[48] Similar mounds are prominent in Pilot Mound Township in Fillmore County. They result from a thick layer of sandstone, called the St. Peter Sandstone, sandwiched between the Decorah Shale layer above and the Shakopee Formation limestone below.[49] When the sandstone is exposed, it erodes rapidly down to the lower limestone layer; however, if the upper layer of limestone or shale is preserved, it serves as a cap to preserve the thick layer of sandstone beneath it.

2
MESS TO MECCA

"THE CYCLONES," 1883

On July 21, 1883, a tornado followed a line beginning in Spink County, South Dakota, sweeping eastward through Sleepy Eye, New Ulm, Mankato and Waseca. It caused a train to derail in Owatonna. In Olmsted County, it struck Kalmar, Cascade, Oronoco and Haverhill Townships, leaving one dead, twenty seriously injured and twenty families homeless. It caused greater damage in Wabasha County, destroying the town of Elgin and killing one and injuring several.

Rochester was unscathed by the first, but exactly one month later, on August 21, 1883, a tornado that would now be a class EF5 began a few miles southwest of Dodge Center at 6:30 p.m., killing five in Dodge County, including the fireman of a train it derailed. It swept through Salem, Kalmar, Cascade and Rochester Townships, destroying buildings and crops, with no deaths in those townships. It touched down and damaged the Stoppel house and barn. It swept over the hill where the Rochester Golf and Country Club is now and continued into town just after 7:00 p.m. Eaton's description is most vivid:

> [A] *slight shower of rain passed over, and for a few moments succeeding, the air was as still as a tomb. Soon light, fleecy clouds were seen scudding athwart the sky at lightning speed, the great dark mass in the west assumed a greenish cast, the heavens blazed with pale yellow lightning, and soon a roar was heard that caused stern faces to blanch and brave hearts to throb with terror. In a moment the storm was upon us. With a roar like ten thousand demons, it*

AMONG THE RUINS.
MINNESOTA.—SCENES IN THE CITY OF ROCHESTER AFTER THE TORNADO OF AUGUST 21ST.
FROM A PHOTO. BY ELMER & TENNEY.—SEE PAGE 38.

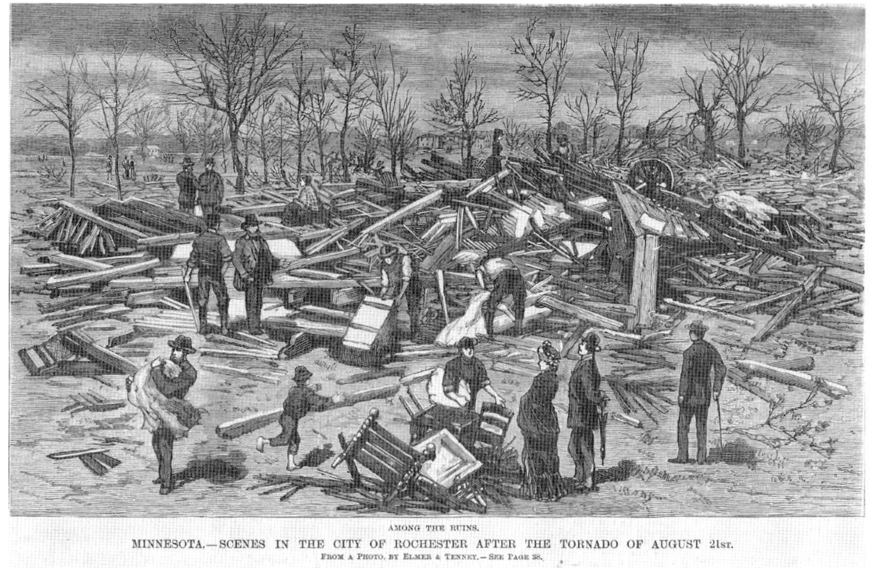

Devastation from tornado. *From* Frank Leslie's Illustrated Newspaper.

> *swept down upon the beautiful city. Like a great coiling serpent, darting out a thousand tongues of lightning, with a hiss like the seething, roaring Niagara, it wrapped the city in its hideous coils. The crashing of buildings and the despairing shrieks of men, women and children were drowned in its terrible roar. An hour later, the pale moonbeams fell upon two hundred ruined homes, two score of dead, ghastly faces, and the stillness of night that was broken by the moans of the wounded and dying. What tongue or pen can half describe this terrible scene of desolation and death?*[50]

It struck first at the top of College Hill (Fourth Street Southwest) and coursed through downtown, destroying the cupola of the courthouse, knocking off steeples from several churches, destroying one brick grocery, ripping the tin roofs from most of the downtown buildings and extensively damaging grain elevators, mills and the Chicago and Northwestern train yard. It destroyed the railroad bridge across the Zumbro and the North Broadway bridge. Because the clouds were so threatening, most of downtown had been evacuated before the storm struck, so despite all of the structural damage downtown, there were no deaths there. That was not the case in Lower Town, the residential neighborhood north of downtown, extending to the North Broadway river crossing. The vortex reached maximum intensity there, over half a mile wide, and moved very slowly, looping back on itself as it scoured the area. Lower

Town was nearly completely leveled, with 135 houses completely destroyed and 200 more damaged. Twenty-six people were killed outright, and over two hundred were injured. At least five died later of injuries. The storm carried on through Haverhill, Viola and Quincy Townships, killing two more, injuring several and destroying many structures and crops. Several bodies were unidentifiable, and several others were taken by families before full accounting. The total deaths were reported to be between thirty-one and thirty-nine, but those are thought to be underestimates.

The power of the Rochester storm was demonstrated by curious observations, such as a wooden plank driven through a small tree, grass straws driven through pieces of wood, a book that was discovered 30 miles from its origin and a $100 certificate of deposit that landed 110 miles away. Trees that were left standing in Lower Town were stripped of leaves and bark.[51] According to the National Weather Service, "Will Reicke was picked up by the tornado, hurled across the Zumbro River and deposited near the Oak Wood Cemetery, where all the gravestones had been blown flat. He escaped with a broken leg, a fractured wrist, and minor injuries."[52]

Two other tornados struck Olmsted County the same day. One was near Pleasant Grove at 3:30 p.m., killing two and injuring ten more in a three-mile path. The other struck between Chatfield and Lewiston at 8:30 p.m., killing one and injuring several more.

The Mayo brothers barely escaped injury. Will was a recent graduate of the University of Michigan Medical School, and Charlie had not yet entered medical school. They were planning to practice eye surgery using the head of a sheep from a slaughterhouse across the river north of Lower Town. When they arrived at the slaughterhouse, they were warned of the approaching storm and headed home. They were on Broadway at Zumbro Street (what is now Second Street South) when the storm struck, blowing the stone cornice off the four-story Cook Hotel and smashing the front of their horse carriage but sparing their lives. They assisted in the relief efforts for the injured, which were directed by their father, W.W. Mayo. The senior Dr. Mayo recruited the Sisters of St. Francis, a local teaching order, to assist in the care of the injured, which, in the absence of a hospital, was set up in the Hotel Rommel on South Broadway.

Generous relief was provided by communities and individuals, most notably the cities of Chicago, Minneapolis, St. Paul, Winona, Saint Cloud and Stillwater, each of which gave large cash contributions. They were sufficient to provide assistance to 233 families; 106 were assisted with rebuilding and 69 with repairing their homes.

St. Marys Hospital, Mother Alfred and W.W. Mayo, 1889

Mother Alfred Moes founded the Third Order of St. Francis, a teaching order of Catholic sisters or nuns. They lived in a convent and staffed a girls' academy (Our Lady of Lourdes) on what is now Center Street. Not long after disaster relief for the tornado was completed, she approached Dr. W.W. Mayo with a proposal to build a hospital. She offered to raise the funds to build the hospital and offered her sisters as staff if Dr. Mayo and his two sons would provide physician staffing. His initial response was negative. He thought, as did most people at the time, that Rochester was too small to support a hospital. It was commonly believed that hospitals were merely a place to die. The practice of performing surgery in a hospital was not yet established. Dr. Mayo, like most of his contemporaries, performed his surgical procedures in patients' homes. Antiseptic practices had not yet been established. Mother Alfred was persistent. She persuaded him to agree to provide medical staffing if she was successful in raising the funds. No one knows the degree to which he was surprised that she was successful in raising the necessary funds ($40,000). Once it was certain that the hospital would be built, the Drs. Mayo made serious study of the current state of the art in hospital architecture and the latest and best design and amenities to build a modern surgical practice.

Construction began in August 1888. Built on nine acres of land on Zumbro Street (Second Street Southwest) just past the city limits, west of downtown, the original structure was forty by sixty feet, three stories, redbrick and stone, with one operating room on the second floor. Scheduled to open on October 1, 1889, it actually opened the day before to allow Dr. Charlie Mayo to perform urgent surgery on a patient with a malignant tumor of the eye. He was assisted by his brother and his father and used an operating table that he built himself.

Six Sisters of St. Francis provided staffing in the first year of operation. They were a teaching order, untrained in nursing. A professional nurse, Edith Graham (later Mayo), trained the sisters in the necessary nursing skills. They worked sixteen- to twenty-hour days and provided all patient care, cleaning, laundry and other services, plus they cooked the food using crops and livestock that they grew on the property. From the beginning, the hospital admitted patients without regard to religion, sex, race or economic circumstances. A year after the opening, Mother Alfred was relieved of her leadership and reassigned to teach in St. Paul by Archbishop John Ireland.

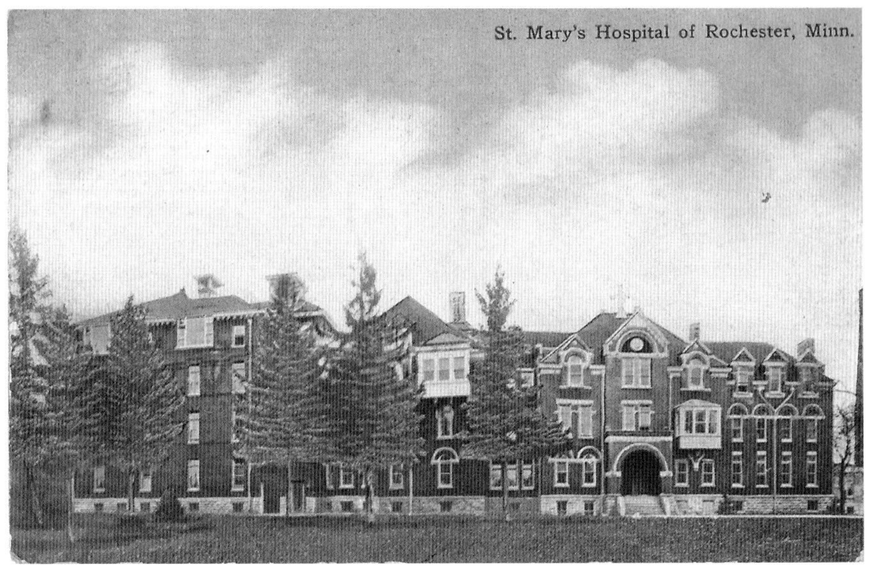

Postcard of St. Marys Hospital, original entrance, with multiple additions.

This has been attributed to complaints from the sisters who preferred teaching to nursing. I wonder how much might have been due to the male hierarchy's distaste for a strong-willed woman. Mother Alfred had previously been similarly relieved of her leadership role among the order of Franciscan sisters that she founded in Joliet, Illinois.

W.W. Mayo was Episcopalian, though an agnostic. It was highly unusual for the time that he joined forces with a Catholic order of sisters to establish a Catholic hospital. Although the hospital accepted patients of all denominations from its beginnings, there was anti-Catholic pushback from part of the community. In response, a competing hospital, Riverside Hospital, was established downtown on Zumbro (Second) Street, east of Broadway. It opened in November 1892, under the leadership of a homeopath, Dr. W.A. Allen. After a flurry of anti-Catholic sentiment directed at St. Marys and the Mayos, Riverside closed unceremoniously in September 1895.[53]

W.W. Mayo was seventy years old when St. Marys opened. He immediately assumed a senior status relative to his sons. When Augustus Stinchfield was hired in 1892, W.W. Mayo retired at age seventy-three.

For nearly one hundred years, the administrative leadership of St. Marys was provided by the Sisters of Saint Francis. These talented, hardworking women were the leaders: Mother Alfred Moes (1889–90), Sister Hyacinth (1890–92), Sister Joseph Dempsey (1892–1939), Sister

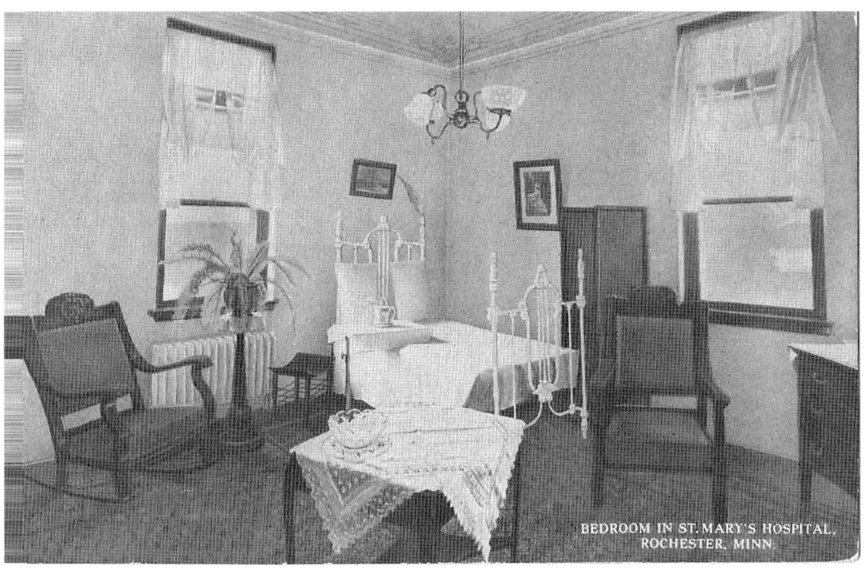

Postcard of St. Marys Hospital, patient room.

Domitilla DuRocher (1939–49), Sister Mary Brigh Cassidy (1949–71) and Sister Generose Gervais (1971–86).

In addition to her remarkable forty-seven-year tenure as administrator, Sister Joseph was Dr. Will's first assistant for twenty-five years, described Sister Joseph's node,[54] among other observations, and started the St. Marys School of Nursing in 1906. She died in 1939, the same year as both Mayo brothers.

After 1971, the apostrophe was deleted from "St. Marys" at the insistence of Sister Generose. According to Sister Ramona Miller, congregational president of the Sisters of St. Francis, "It was an important spelling promoted by Sister Generose Gervais….She opposed using the apostrophe because it conveyed a possessive meaning, and she said that the hospital did not belong to Saint Mary."[55]

In addition to the succession of administrators and staff, there was a succession of additions and new buildings as the surgical and then medical practice grew. The hospital opened in 1889 with 27 beds, plus 18 emergency beds. It had very limited equipment and supplies, including an elevator shaft with no elevator. It served an exclusively surgical population. The Mayo's surgical practice grew so rapidly that additions were required in 1893, 1898 and 1903, reaching a capacity of 150 beds. Another addition in 1909 doubled capacity to 300 beds. A new surgical building (later renamed the Joseph Building) added in July 1922 increased bed capacity to 650. The Tower and

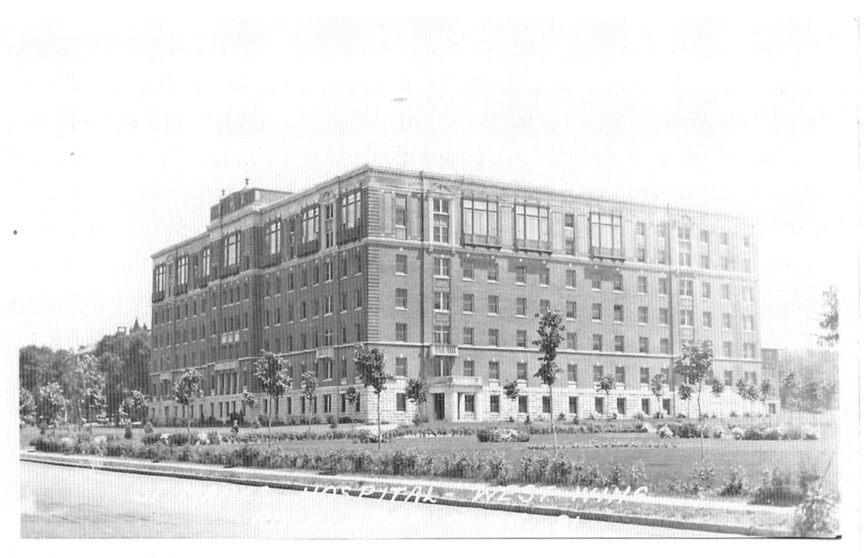

Postcard of St. Marys Hospital, Joseph Building, 1922.

Francis Buildings were added in 1941, raising total beds to 850. The Domitilla Building opened in 1956. The Alfred Building raised the total number of beds to 1,020 in 1967. The Mary Brigh Building opened in 1980. It is a huge complex with multiple segments and up to ten floors—100,000 square feet per floor, 43 operating rooms on lower floors, 6 nursing units per floor, 12 ICU beds per unit (or more beds if lower acuity) and a heliport on top.

The construction of the Alfred and Mary Brigh buildings necessitated the demolition of part of the Marion Hall nurses' quarters and the beautiful (some say acoustically perfect) auditorium that was located on the current site of the Mary Brigh Building.

The Generose (Psychiatry) Building opened in 1993 with three floors and 270,000 square feet of space. A 2019 addition to Generose added three floors with 150,000 square feet to house the Physical Medicine and Rehabilitation inpatient service. The most recent building, named in honor of publishing magnate and philanthropist John M. Nasseff, has eleven stories with 430,000 square feet of space. Each floor can accommodate up to 24 beds. It currently holds 162 beds, dedicated mostly to cardiology.

It is rarely noted that during a large portion of the careers of the Mayo brothers, there was no Mayo Clinic, per se, since the first building called Mayo Clinic opened in 1914, twenty-five years after the opening of St. Marys Hospital.

In 1986, it was clear that Mayo Clinic and its two affiliated hospitals could function more efficiently as a single legal entity. To achieve that, the Sisters of St. Francis and the Rochester Methodist Hospital board transferred ownership of their two respective hospitals to Mayo Clinic. The sisters asked to have an enduring Franciscan presence in the management of the hospital. That is provided by the Mayo Clinic Values Council, whose mission is to "promote the Mayo Clinic Values across all of Mayo Clinic. The Council will also assist to perpetuate the Franciscan Legacy on the Saint Marys Campus and across all of Mayo Clinic."

Since January 2014, the St. Marys complex has been called Mayo Clinic Hospital, St. Marys Campus. It has 1,265 licensed beds and 70 operating rooms.

My Brother and I

William James "Will" Mayo was born on June 29, 1861, in the Mayo family home in the frontier village of Le Sueur, Minnesota, the fifth child of William Worrall and Louise Abigail (Wright) Mayo. Two siblings died as infants, Horace (1851–1852) and Sarah Frances (1859–1860). His two surviving sisters were Gertrude Emily Berkman (1853–1938) and Phoebe Louise (1856–1885). His brother, Charles Horace "Charlie," was born on July 19, 1865, in the Mayo family home in Rochester on Franklin Street (First Avenue Southwest), the site of the 1914 Mayo Clinic Building, and currently the Siebens Building.

Both brothers attended Central School, across Franklin Street, and received instruction in Latin, art and classics at Sanford Niles's private Rochester Training Academy.[56] Their mother instructed them in botany and astronomy and their father in chemistry, physics, anatomy and medical sciences. They were encouraged to study in their parents' extensive library. Both worked as pharmacy clerks at Geisinger & Newton's Drug Store. Both assisted their father's medical practice, helping at the office and on house calls. They performed minor procedures, such as suturing, and even administered anesthesia while their father operated. They also performed autopsies. Both attributed their career choice to growing up in that environment. Dr. Will recalled, "We were reared in medicine as a farmer boy is reared in farming."[57]

Though close throughout their lives and their professional careers, the brothers had very different personalities. Growing up, Will was academically

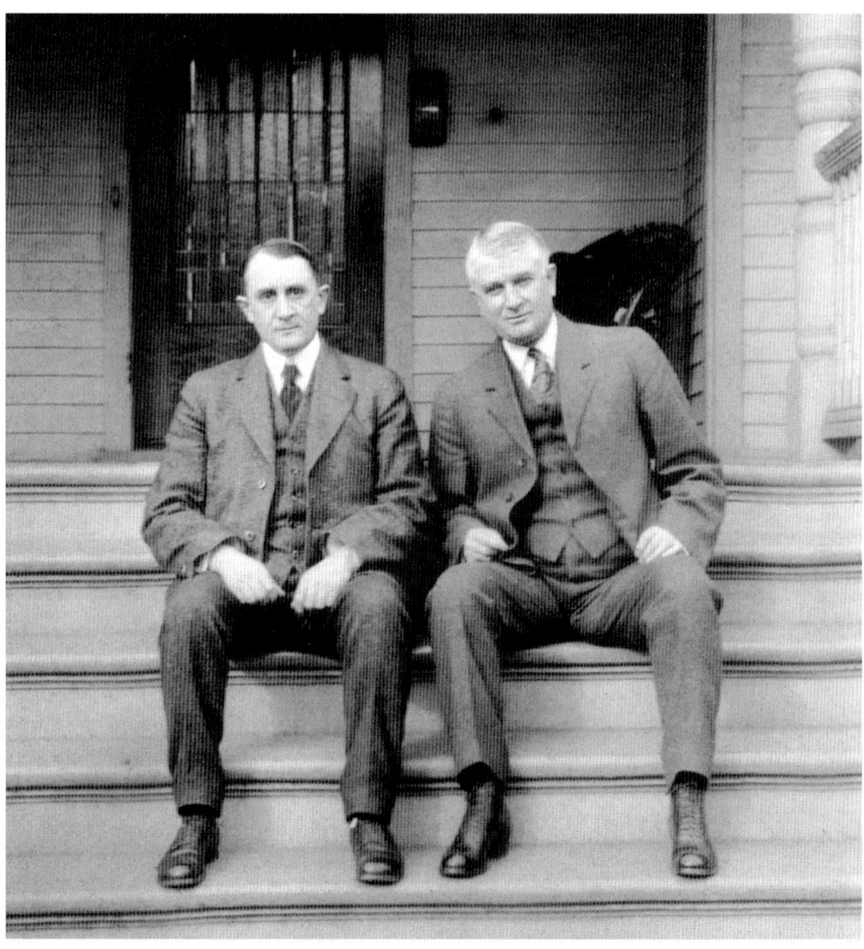

Mayo brothers on Dr. Will's (*right*) front step. *By permission of Mayo Foundation for Medical Education and Research.*

inclined and disliked farm chores but loved assisting in their father's medical practice. Charlie was less academically inclined, mischievous in school and a poor speller but loved working and spending time on the family farm. He was mechanically inclined and could fix anything. At fourteen, he installed the phone to connect the family farm to their father's office. Harry Harwick compared the two as adults: "Doctor Will, a natural leader, was rather reserved, analytical, dominating (though without arrogance), relentless in demanding perfection of himself and others, with an uncanny ability to foresee the future. Dr. Charlie was warm, understanding, wonderfully humorous, possessing the common touch."[58]

Dr. Charlie's son, "Dr. Chuck," wrote: "Uncle Will was the taller, with an aristocratic face and the bearing of a general. My father's posture inclined towards comfort. Uncle Will's clothes had mannequin neatness and fit, while Father could look disheveled in a freshly pressed suit." He described his Uncle Will and his mother "watching Father walking along laughing with two friends. 'Everybody likes Charlie, don't they,' he mused. 'They aren't afraid of him. No one ever puts an arm around my shoulder as they do with him.' Then Uncle Will said brusquely, 'But then, I wouldn't like it if they did.'"[59]

Their love of automobiles was also illustrative. Charlie owned the very first automobile in Rochester, drove them enthusiastically, assembled multiple vehicles himself from parts and served as a dealer for several makes of autos to ensure access to vehicles. Will, by contrast, loved to travel by car but always with the service of a driver. He used chauffeured drives in the country to discuss management decisions with others, particularly administrator Harry Harwick.

Their personality differences persisted throughout their lives, though they were nearly inseparable. Throughout their careers, they maintained a single checking account that each drew from as needed.

Will received his MD from the University of Michigan Medical School on June 28, 1883. Shortly after, he told a family friend, "I expect to remain in Rochester and to become the greatest surgeon in the world."[60] He joined his father in the family practice, which at that point moved from W.W. Mayo's old office on Third Street to the Ramsey Block (or Massey's Building) offices at the southeast corner of Zumbro and Main Streets (Second Street and First Avenue Southwest). In 1884, Dr. Will married Hattie Marie Damon (1864–1952), a Rochester native. They had five children, of whom two daughters survived infancy, Carrie Louise (1887–1960), who married Dr. Donald Balfour, and Phoebe Gertrude (1897–1994), who married Dr. Waltman Walters. Both of their husbands were Mayo Clinic physicians.

Charlie received his MD from Chicago Medical School (later known as Northwestern University Medical School) in 1888. He returned to Rochester and joined his father and older brother in the family medical practice. Edith Graham was a native of Rochester. She received her training as a professional nurse in Chicago and was recruited by W.W. Mayo to serve in the Mayo practice and St. Marys Hospital as a professionally trained nurse, nurse educator for the Sisters of St. Francis and nurse anesthetist. She married Dr. Charlie in 1893. Together they had eight children, six of whom survived childhood: Margaret (1895), Dorothy (1897–1960), Charles William "Chuck" (1898–1968), Edith "Missy" Mayo Rankin (1900–1982), Joseph Graham "Joe," (1902–1936), Louise Mayo (Trenholm) Elwinger

(1905–1993), Rachel (1908–1910) and Esther Mayo Hartzell (1909–1971), plus two adopted children, John Hartley Nelson (1911–1972) and Marilynn M. "Sally" Mayo (1920–1984). Charles William "Chuck" Mayo and Joseph Graham Mayo were both staff surgeons at the clinic. Dr. Joe Mayo was killed at the age of thirty-four in November 1936, when a train struck his car. His dog Foosie was killed in the accident and was buried with him in the same casket. Dr. Chuck was also killed in an auto accident on his seventieth birthday in 1968. Charlie's grandson Charles Horace Mayo II and two great-grandsons, Joseph Graham Mayo III and Chester "Chet" Wilson Planck Mayo, trained as residents at the clinic.

In 1892, W.W. Mayo recruited Augustus Stinchfield, a successful practitioner in Eyota, to join the Mayo practice in Rochester. Once Stinchfield was on board, W.W. Mayo retired from the practice at age seventy-three. Others who were invited to be partners in the firm included Christopher Graham (Edith Graham Mayo's brother), E. Starr Judd, Henry S. Plummer, Melvin Millet and Donald Balfour. The Mayos encouraged, and the group embraced, the concept of specialization as it evolved, thus they invented the integrated multi-specialty group practice.

The Mayo brothers grew their surgical practice as they increasingly specialized in surgery. Dr. Will concentrated on abdominal and gynecological procedures. In contrast, Dr. Charlie was a remarkably versatile surgeon who could do practically any type of surgery. He developed his skills in a broader range, including ophthalmologic surgery; ear, nose and throat; thyroid surgery; neurosurgery; peripheral vascular and orthopedic surgery. Both brothers were early adopters of "Listerism," or the use of sterile techniques to reduce operative infections. They traveled frequently to learn new procedures developed by colleagues in the United States and Europe. They both devised surgical instruments to facilitate improved techniques. They encouraged their colleagues to do likewise.

Dr. Will quickly developed his talent as a public speaker. He excelled at it and had tremendous surgical results to report, both in terms of numbers and outcomes. Dr. Charlie was a hesitant speaker. He had similarly superlative results, but he did not gravitate to public speaking. He had a circuitous and long-winded speaking style. His wife, Edith, worked with him to improve his technique. They rehearsed his speeches together, and she often gave him feedback from the audience during his speeches. As his speaking technique improved, he became popular for his conversational and jocular style. Dr. Will gave his most famous speech to the graduating class of Rush Medical College in 1910. He stated:

> *As we grow in learning, we more justly appreciate our dependence upon each other. The sum-total of medical knowledge is now so great and wide-spreading that it would be futile for one man to attempt to acquire, or for any one man to assume that he has, even a good working knowledge of any large part of the whole. The very necessities of the case are driving practitioners into cooperation. The best interest of the patient is the only interest to be considered, and in order that the sick may have the benefit of advancing knowledge, union of forces is necessary.*[61]

Both brothers served as president of the American Medical Association, Dr. Will in 1906–7 and Dr. Charlie in 1917–18. In addition, Dr. Will served as president of the Minnesota State Medical Society in 1894. In 1907, he was appointed to the Board of Regents of the University of Minnesota, a position he continued until 1939. He was president of the Society for Clinical Surgery in 1911 and president of the American Surgical Association in 1913. Dr. Charlie served on the Rochester School Board and as Olmsted County public health director. He was a regent and later president of the American College of Surgeons, president of the Minnesota Medical Association in 1906 and president of the American Surgical Association in 1931. Throughout their careers, when Dr. Will received an award or accolade, he usually accepted "on behalf of my brother and I." It was said jokingly that if he were elected president of the United States, he would take the oath of office "on behalf of my brother and I." Both were Freemasons of the Rochester Lodge and the Grand Lodge of Minnesota, and they were active in other many other civic and social clubs.

Post-graduate medical education evolved in Rochester, beginning with the Surgeons' Club (see the next section). When George Vincent became president of the University of Minnesota in 1911, he quickly became aware of the educational activities in Rochester and encouraged the Mayos to affiliate with the university and develop research programs and formal post-graduate medical education. A limitation to the relationship was the fact that the Mayos' organization was a private partnership. To provide organization support for academic affiliation, Mayo Foundation for Medical Education and Research was incorporated on February 8, 1915, executed by Drs. Will and Charlie Mayo, Christopher Graham, Henry Plummer, E. Starr Judd and Donald C. Balfour. The Mayo brothers endowed the foundation with $1.5 million from their personal fortune and promised to pay foundation expenses until the endowment plus dividends totaled $2.0 million.

The proposed affiliation of the university with Mayo Foundation drew opposition, primarily from medical faculty of the university and private physicians in the Twin Cities. Hennepin and Ramsey County Medical Societies passed resolutions denouncing the proposed affiliation. Critics accused the Mayos of seeking publicity and financial gain, extracting resources from the university, diverting prestige from the university medical school and so forth. The critics were ridiculed in the national press. A bill banning the affiliation was passed by the state senate but was too late in the session to be addressed by the house. On June 15, 1915, the University Regents unanimously approved the affiliation with Mayo Foundation.

In the next state legislative session in 1917, the bill of opposition was revived. Dr. Will Mayo was asked to address the Senate committee considering the bill on March 15, 1917. The *Minneapolis Morning Tribune* reported his speech, which was extemporaneous and otherwise unrecorded. It is called "The Lost Oration." He explained the background and motivation of the gift. He concluded:

> *I can't understand why all this opposition should have been aroused over the affiliation with the University. It seems to be the idea of some persons that no one can want to do anything for anybody without having some sinister motive back of it. If we wanted money, we have it. That can't be the reason for our offer. We want the money to go back to the people, from whom it came, and we think we can best give it back to them through medical education. Now let's call a spade a spade. This money belongs to the people, and I don't care two raps whether the medical profession of the state like the way this money has been offered for use or not. It wasn't their money. "That these dead shall not have died in vain." That line explains why we want to do this thing. What better could we do than take young men and help them to become proficient in the profession so as to prevent needless deaths?*[62]

He received thunderous applause for his speech, and the bill died in committee.[63] The endowment reached $2 million in 1934. On February 15, 1934, the Mayos transferred another $500,000 to the endowment.

Drs. Will and Charlie Mayo both served with distinction in the army during World War I (1914–18). They alternated with each other to cover duties in Rochester, managing the clinic and duties in Washington for the war effort. Will served the surgeon general of the U.S. Army as chief adviser for surgical services while Charlie alternated as associate chief adviser. They both served on the Committee of American Physicians for Medical

Preparedness, Will as chair. And they served on the General Medical Board of the Council for National Defense, with Will as a member of its executive committee and Charlie as his alternate. Both achieved the rank of colonel during the war and remained in the Army Reserve after the war. They received the Distinguished Service Medal in 1926 and were commissioned as brigadier generals in 1931.

The strain of the war effort affected the health of both brothers. Charlie developed pneumonia, and Will developed hepatitis. The realities of war and illness, particularly Dr. Will's hepatitis, prompted thoughts of succession after the Mayos' time passed. To establish a more durable organization, on October 8, 1919, the Mayo brothers transferred all the assets of Mayo Clinic to the newly created Mayo Properties Association. It was a self-perpetuating charitable organization, so it was tax exempt. The assets included all the buildings, all contents and all other assets of the clinic, which in 1925 was valued at $5.0 million for properties and $5.5 million for securities. The Mayo Properties Association was the brainchild of business manager Harry Harwick and attorney George Granger. It had the support of most of Mayo's partners except one. Dr. Christopher Graham, Dr. Charlie's brother-in-law, refused to sign the agreement. He disapproved of the foundation and would not agree to this transfer to it. He disputed ownership of the assets and the ethics of tax avoidance. When no compromise could be found, he was forced to resign from the group (and retired from the practice of medicine), causing distress in the family. As a final step, in 1923, the clinic was reorganized as a "voluntary association" in which all staff, including the original partners of the firm, were salaried employees.

On July 1, 1928, at the age of sixty-seven, Dr. Will returned to his office from a morning of operating at St. Marys. He appeared depressed. His secretary asked what the matter was. He said, "I've just done my last operation." Without explanation, he never operated again. Years later, he said that he felt he had lost the mental flexibility needed to handle the stress of operating,[64] and Dr. Chuck, in his autobiography, said that Dr. Will had developed a tremor.[65] Dr. Charlie continued operating for a year and a half, until he suffered a retinal hemorrhage followed by a series of strokes. They continued to consult and advise their younger colleagues. In November 1932, Dr. Will announced that the following month both Drs. Mayo and Dr. Plummer would relinquish their positions on the Board of Governors to be replaced by younger staff members, thus completing the transition of power from the Mayo Clinic founders to their younger colleagues. The brothers continued traveling in retirement, now able to travel together without needing to keep one at home to manage the clinic. Dr. Charlie no longer tolerated Minnesota winters, so they wintered thereafter at homes in Tucson, Arizona.

The brothers died within two months of each other. Dr. Charlie died of pneumonia on May 26, 1939, in Chicago at the age of seventy-three. Dr. Will died in Rochester on July 28, 1939, at age seventy-eight, of gastric carcinoma. Ironically, that tumor had been a major emphasis in his surgical practice. They are buried at the family plot at Oakwood Cemetery on either side of their parents and next to their wives. Sister Joseph died the same year. The crisis of transition that might have resulted was prevented by the orderly transfer of management that they organized and executed.

THE SURGEONS' CLUB

Post-graduate medical education is arguably the key, or one of the main keys, to the success of the Mayos, beginning with W.W. Mayo. He and his sons traveled frequently to learn new medical knowledge, particularly new surgical techniques. Early on, despite their frontier location, the Mayos welcomed visitors, local practitioners as well as visitors from afar, to observe their practice. The number of visitors grew throughout their careers. By 1906, the number of daily observers grew to twenty to forty per day. To manage the crowds, the visitors self-organized and created the International Surgeons' Club, later shortened to the Surgeons' Club at the request of Dr. Will, who thought the original name was ostentatious. In 1919, the name was changed to the Physicians' and Surgeons' Club. The club charged a small membership fee, which was used to rent space in the Masonic Lodge on the floor above the Mayo partners' medical offices. The visiting physicians observed the Mayos and their colleagues operating in the morning. In the afternoon, they discussed cases downtown and used their time for reading and further discussion. When the Mayo Graduate School of Medicine was formed in 1915, the functions of the Surgeons' Club gradually merged with the Graduate School and the Mayo Alumni Association. The early emphasis on post-graduate medical education persists to this day, as indicated by the fact that Mayo Clinic Alix School of Medicine is one of the smallest medical schools in the country (the motto is *Non multa sed bona*, "Not many, but good"), whereas Mayo Clinic School of Graduate Medical Education is one of the largest programs of post-graduate medical education in the world.

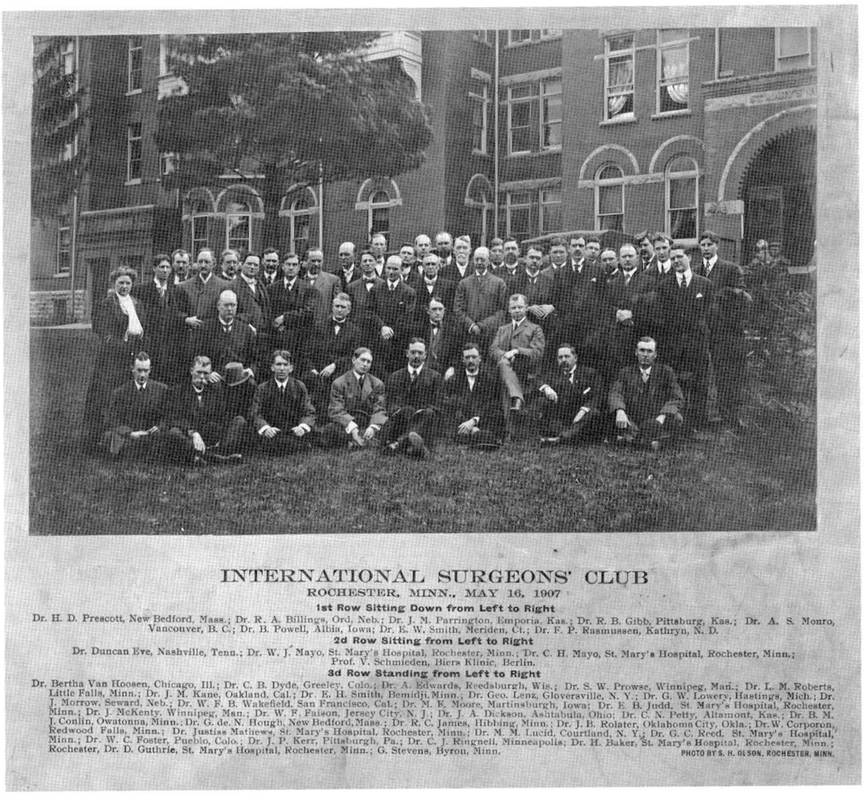

INTERNATIONAL SURGEONS' CLUB
ROCHESTER, MINN., MAY 16, 1907
1st Row Sitting Down from Left to Right
Dr. H. D. Prescott, New Bedford, Mass.; Dr. R. A. Billings, Ord, Neb.; Dr. J. M. Parrington, Emporia, Kas.; Dr. R. B. Gibb, Pittsburg, Kas.; Dr. A. S. Monro, Vancouver, B. C.; Dr. B. Powell, Albia, Iowa; Dr. E. W. Smith, Meriden, Ct.; Dr. F. P. Rasmussen, Kathryn, N. D.
2d Row Sitting from Left to Right
Dr. Duncan Eve, Nashville, Tenn.; Dr. W. J. Mayo, St. Mary's Hospital, Rochester, Minn.; Dr. C. H. Mayo, St. Mary's Hospital, Rochester, Minn.; Prof. V. Schmieden, Biers Klinic, Berlin.
3d Row Standing from Left to Right
Dr. Bertha Van Hoosen, Chicago, Ill.; Dr. C. B. Dyde, Greeley, Colo.; Dr. A. Edwards, Reedsburgh, Wis.; Dr. S. W. Prowse, Winnipeg, Man.; Dr. L. M. Roberts, Little Falls, Minn.; Dr. J. M. Kane, Oakland, Cal.; Dr. E. H. Smith, Bemidji, Minn.; Dr. Geo. Lenz, Gloversville, N. Y.; Dr. G. W. Lowery, Hastings, Mich.; Dr. J. Morrow, Seward, Neb.; Dr. W. F. B. Wakefield, San Francisco, Cal.; Dr. M. F. Moore, Martinsburgh, Iowa; Dr. E. B. Judd, St. Mary's Hospital, Rochester, Minn.; Dr. J. McKenty, Winnipeg, Man.; Dr. W. F. Faison, Jersey City, N. J.; Dr. J. A. Dickson, Ashtabula, Ohio; Dr. C. N. Petty, Altamont, Kas.; Dr. B. M. J. Conlin, Owatonna, Minn.; Dr. G. de. N. Hough, New Bedford, Mass.; Dr. R. C. James, Hibbing, Minn.; Dr. J. B. Rolater, Oklahoma City, Okla.; Dr. W. Corporon, Redwood Falls, Minn.; Dr. Justiss Mathews, St. Mary's Hospital, Rochester, Minn.; Dr. M. M. Lucid, Courtland, N. Y.; Dr. G. C. Reed, St. Mary's Hospital, Minn.; Dr. W. C. Foster, Pueblo, Colo.; Dr. J. P. Kerr, Pittsburgh, Pa.; Dr. C. J. Ringnell, Minneapolis; Dr. H. Baker, St. Mary's Hospital, Rochester, Minn.; Rochester, Dr. D. Guthrie, St. Mary's Hospital, Rochester, Minn.; G. Stevens, Byron, Minn.
PHOTO BY S. H. OLSON, ROCHESTER, MINN.

International Surgeons' Club, 1907.

Nursing Education

The history of nursing education in Rochester is a story of dualities: St. Marys and Methodist/Kahler/Colonial, hospital-based nursing programs and programs based in educational institutions, certificate programs and degree programs, associate and baccalaureate programs, the Minnesota State College system and the University of Minnesota, undergraduate and graduate programs.

Excellent medical care is not achievable without excellent nursing care. When St. Marys Hospital opened in 1889, the Sisters of St. Francis staffed the hospital, with nursing education provided on the job by Edith Graham (Mayo). The sisters worked extraordinary hours, but as the Mayo surgical practice grew relentlessly, it was apparent that the sisters were outnumbered. In a small town, there was no supply of trained nurses to recruit to the hospital, so Sister

Joseph Dempsey, the hospital administrator, recognized that the only solution was to start a school of nursing. St. Marys Hospital Training School for Nurses opened in November 1906, directed by Anna Jamme, initially as a two-year program. It grew to a three-year program in 1914–16, with Mary Ledwidge as superintendent of nurses. The school was first accredited by the state in April 1916. During World War II, through the U.S. Cadet Nurse Corps, 42 Japanese American women were freed from the Japanese internment camps to study nursing at the St. Marys program.[66] The diploma program was replaced by an associate degree program with Rochester State Junior College in 1967. St. Marys School of Nursing closed after the class of 1970, having produced a total of 3,865 graduates over the sixty-five years of education, nearly 60 per year. A school of psychiatric nurses training operated at the Rochester State Hospital from 1892 to 1968.

The downtown hospital system evolved somewhat later. The need for trained nurses was even more quickly apparent because of World War I. Colonial Hospital opened in 1916, and the Kahler Corporation was formed in 1917. The Colonial Hospital Training School of Nurses opened as a one-year training program in April 1918, directed by Mary J. Gill, superintendent of nurses at Colonial, and Dr. Melvin Henderson, chief of staff of Colonial Hospital. Military training was planned to follow the first year but was canceled after Armistice Day (November 11, 1918). The program expanded to two years in 1919 and then three years in 1920, achieving professional diploma status. In 1921, the school was renamed the Kahler Hospitals School of Nursing. The school grew enormously to 473 students under the Cadet Nurses Corps Program during World War II. After the war, the economics of for-profit hospitals became increasingly unfavorable until 1954, when the nonprofit Rochester Methodist Hospital was created and the hospitals and their programs were transferred and renamed. The school became the Methodist-Kahler School of Nursing. It closed after the class of 1970, with 3,827 total diploma graduates, just over 73 graduates per year.

Since 1970, nursing programs in Rochester have been sponsored by educational institutions. Rochester Junior College, which became Rochester Community and Technical College in 1996, has provided LPN and associate degree RN programs. Winona State University has provided a baccalaureate RN program. Most recently, the University of Minnesota has developed a Rochester campus with an emphasis in health sciences. They provide a baccalaureate RN program.

Post-baccalaureate nursing education includes many options. In addition to masters and doctoral level programs available through the University of

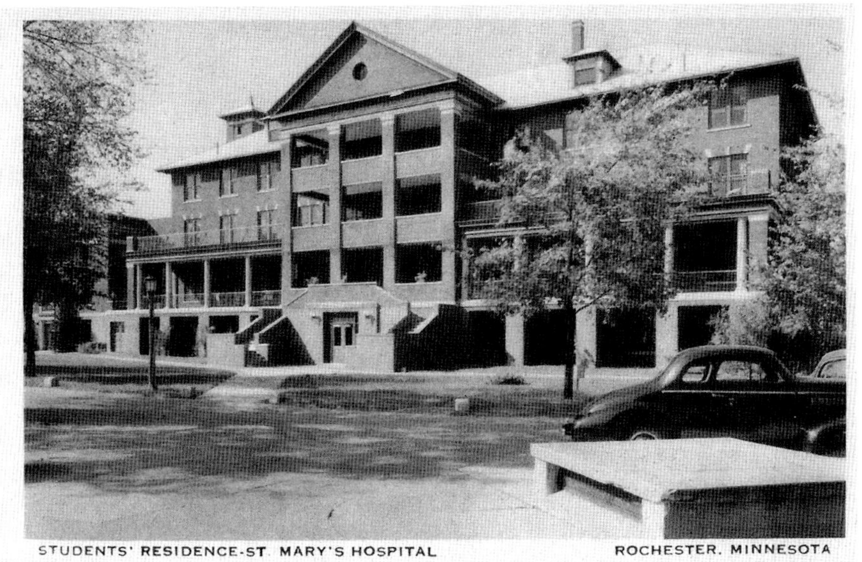

Postcard of Marion Hall, nursing students' dormitory at St. Marys.

Minnesota and Winona State University, other institutions provide additional options, some online exclusively or with low-residence requirements. Options for training and certification for nurse practitioners, nurse anesthetists and other advanced practice nurses round out the options.

The Mayo Clinic nurse anesthesia program, and the practice of nurse-administered anesthesia, began in 1889, making it the oldest continuously operating program for nurse anesthesia in existence. In that year, Dr. William Worrall Mayo began training Edith Graham (Mayo), followed by her successor, Alice Magaw. Magaw was the sole anesthetist for Dr. Will and Dr. Charlie Mayo from 1893 to 1900 and was renowned for masterful technique and gentle touch. She reportedly administered anesthesia to fourteen thousand surgical patients without a single anesthesia-related death. The practice at Mayo contrasted with academic medical centers, where interns were assigned the task with no training. Unsurprisingly, better results were achieved by Mayo's professional nurse anesthetists. Nurse anesthetists continue to play a large role in the procedural practice at Mayo Clinic.[67]

In 2016, Mayo Clinic Rochester was awarded Magnet Recognition by the American Nurses Association for the fifth time, one of only six health care organizations to be so recognized. Magnet status is considered the highest recognition achievable for nursing excellence.[68]

THE QUEEN CITY V. MED CITY

Rochester's nickname, the "Queen City," originated with an ad for Delbert Darling's Business College and Photographic Institute in 1879. No one has ever come up with a specific regal rationale for the name. It was used over the years by a number of businesses and organizations, including Queen City Band, Queen City Bottling Works, Queen City Cafeteria, Queen City Candy Co., Queen City Cigar Co., Queen City Creamery Co., Queen City Decorators, Queen City Dray Line, Queen City Finance, Queen City Gun Club, Queen City Mills, Queen City Monument Co., Queen City Motors, Queen City Nursery, Queen City Oil Co., Queen City Orchestra and Queen City Silver Fox Farms.

The nickname has faded somewhat in recent years but remains a popular topic among local history buffs. Recently, there has been some renewed interest. Current Queen City users include Queen City Coffee & Juice at the Castle, Queen City Construction Inc., Queen City Center and Queen City Panel.[69]

The more contemporary nickname, "Med City," might have greater recognition and relevance. That name originated with the Med City Marathon beginning in 1996.[70] Other current users include Med City Animal Hospital, Med City Beat, Med City Collision, Med City Dental,

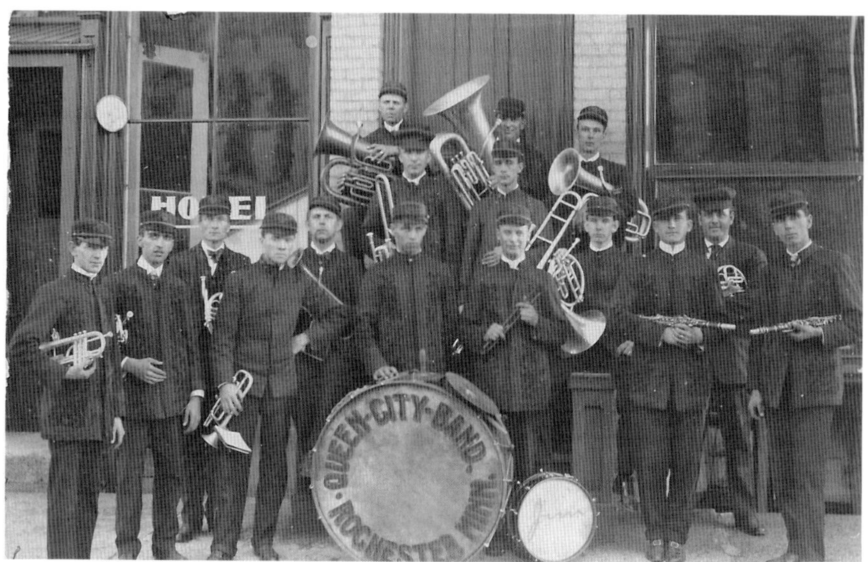

Postcard of the Queen City Band, 1902.

Med City Driving School, Med City FC (men's soccer), Med City Freeze (men's football), Med City Mobility, Med City Nutrition, Med City Taxi and Med City Vapors.

Schuster Brewery

Among the most attractive and highly valued postcards from Rochester were those produced for the Schuster Brewery. A single-bottle version and two double-bottle versions exist. Henry Schuster, the founder, was a native of Prussia, born in 1835. He came to Rochester in 1863 and three years later bought a brewery that he expanded. In 1871, a fire destroyed the business, but he rebuilt it and successfully expanded business until his early death in 1885. His two young sons, Henry Jr. and Frederick, inherited the business and managed it successfully for many years.

By 1910, Joseph Leonard reported it to be the largest business in Rochester, with fifty employees producing ten million bottles per year. Half was beer

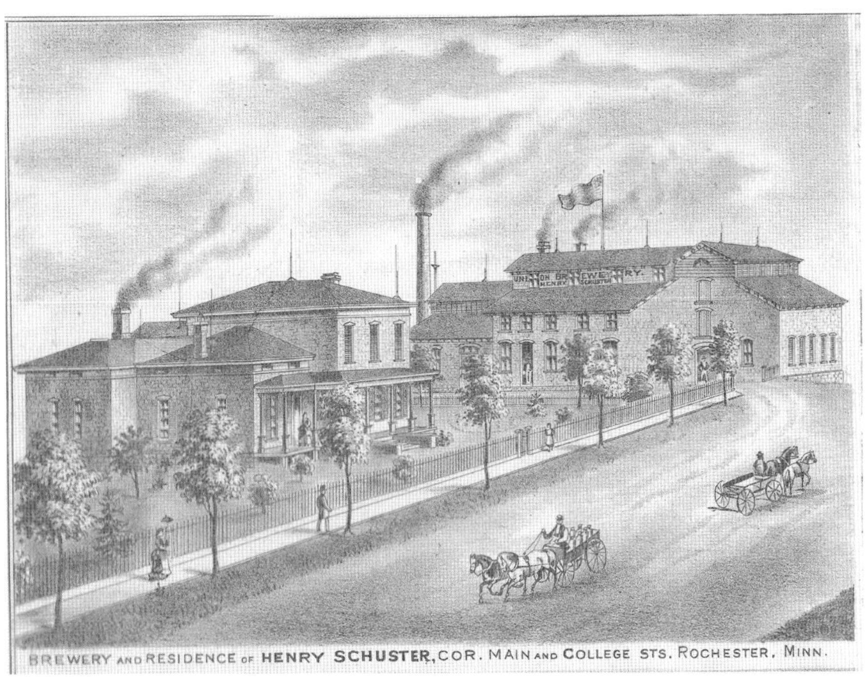

BREWERY AND RESIDENCE OF HENRY SCHUSTER, COR. MAIN AND COLLEGE STS. ROCHESTER, MINN.

Schuster Brewery and residence. *From Andreas's* Historical Atlas of the State of Minnesota, *1874.*

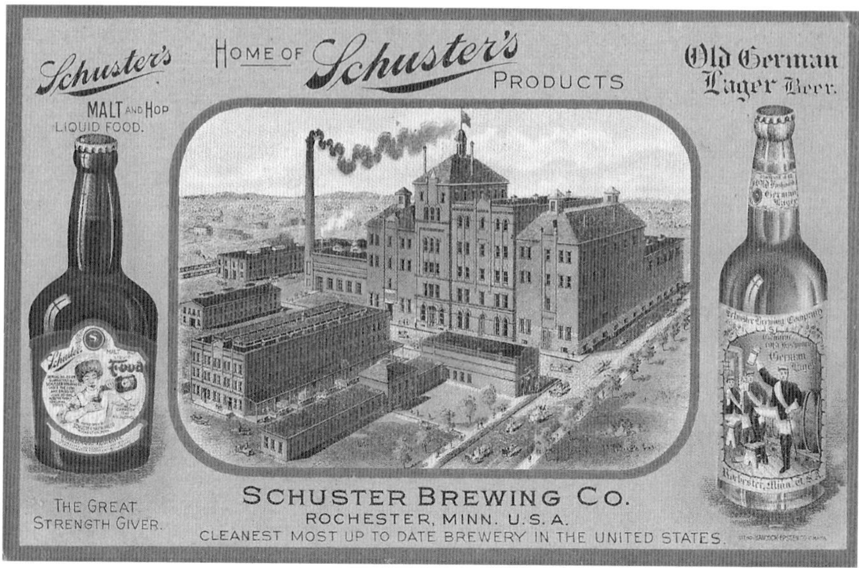

Postcard of Schuster Brewery, circa 1917.

and half "Malt and Hop Liquid Food," a tonic that was sold in drugstores. It contained 4.0 percent alcohol and was very popular. They shipped to twenty-three states. The business covered most of a two-block campus bordered by Fourth and Sixth Streets Southwest and Broadway and First Avenue Southwest.[71] When Prohibition was declared, the brewery modified its output, continuing the malt tonic and switching from beer to a cereal beverage that contained less than 0.5 percent alcohol. Unfortunately, the near beer business was not sufficient to support the large facility. The plant was closed in 1922 and sold to Rochester Dairy in 1925.[72] Fred Schuster transitioned to a successful realtor with extensive dealings with Mayo Clinic and its employees. His son, G. Slade Schuster, a Harvard master's of business administration graduate, was a Mayo Clinic administrator for forty-three years and succeeded Harry Harwick as head of Mayo Clinic Administration from 1952 to 1971.

Fire!

The Rochester Fire Department (RFD) started as a volunteer company on January 22, 1866. The first fire station was completed on October 8, 1870, and was located on the west riverbank at Third Street Southeast, next to the

Olds & Fishback Mill. A Silsby Little Giant portable steam engine pump drew water from the underground mill race and provided water pressure for commercial buildings on Broadway when not fighting fires. Firefighting capabilities increased with underground cisterns in 1874 and, in 1887, the installation of eight miles of water main and 120 hydrants. The second main fire hall was built in 1890 east of the old city hall on Third Street Southwest. Buildings were made more fire resistant over time with better materials, fire extinguishers, alarms and fire suppression systems.

The third central fire station was built in 1898 at the south end of Broadway, just south of the intersection at College Street (Fourth Street). At the time, Broadway ended there and did not cross the Zumbro as it now does south of Sixth Street. The southbound route took a dogleg at College Street (Fourth Street South) over to Dubuque Street (Third Avenue Southeast). The third fire hall was one of the most beautiful buildings in Rochester history. It had a four-face tower clock by Seth Thomas. It was featured in dozens of postcards after the turn of the century, with images of the fire station by itself or as the central figure in various views of South Broadway. In 1912, the first motorized American La France fire pumper was acquired, and in 1917, a seventy-five-foot aerial ladder was added.

When the South Broadway bridge over the Zumbro was built, the extension of Broadway forced the demolition of the third fire hall and the construction in 1930 of the fourth central fire station on South Broadway at Sixth Street. That building was replaced on the same site in 1995–96.

The Seth Thomas Tower Clock was preserved. It was restored in 1982 and placed at the entry to the Rochester Civic Center. Since 2017, it has needed a new home. Prompted by an endowment from local historian Alan Calavano, RFD proposed building a new tower to house the clock and bell. The fire poles from the early fire stations have also been preserved and installed in the current central fire station. A history of RFD was published in 2000.[73]

The Norton Hotel opened in 1914, located at 104 Second Street Southeast, overlooking the Zumbro River on the current site of Fontaine Towers. February 6, 1967, was extremely cold, with a daytime high temperature of negative twelve degrees Fahrenheit. Fire broke out in one of the guest rooms. Battling the fire was made difficult by the extreme cold. The building was a total loss and at the end was encased in icicles, which provided dramatic photographs. Several people were injured evacuating the building, and three tenants died in their rooms. The hotel lacked a sprinkler system, which was used to promote that requirement thereafter.

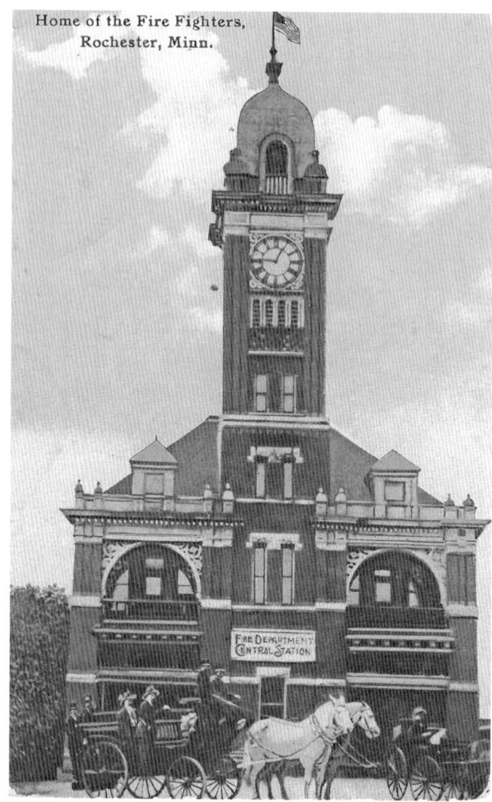

Left: Postcard of Central Fire Station.

Below: Norton Hotel fire aftermath. *Courtesy of the History Center of Olmsted County*.

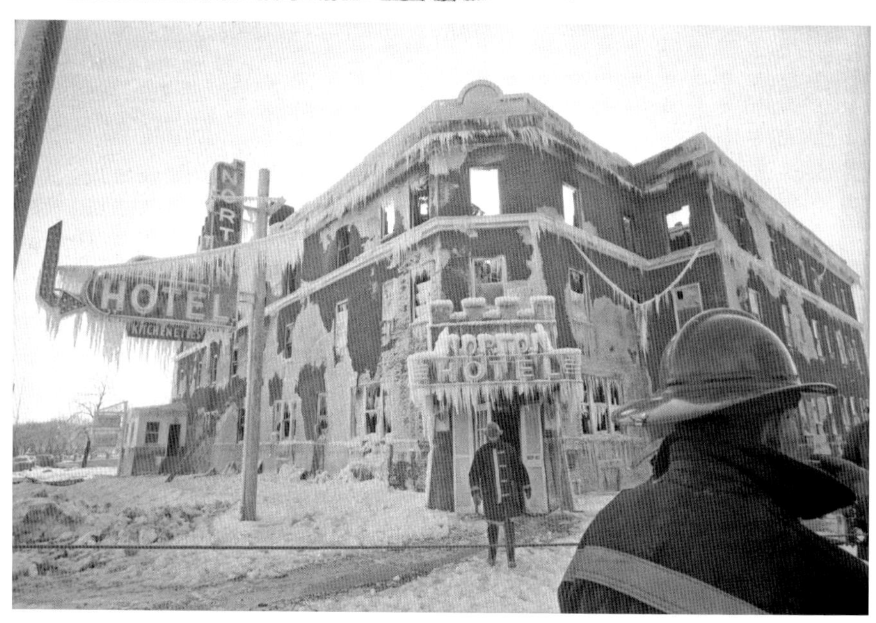

R. R. FIRE JUNE 1, 1910
ROCHESTER, MINN.

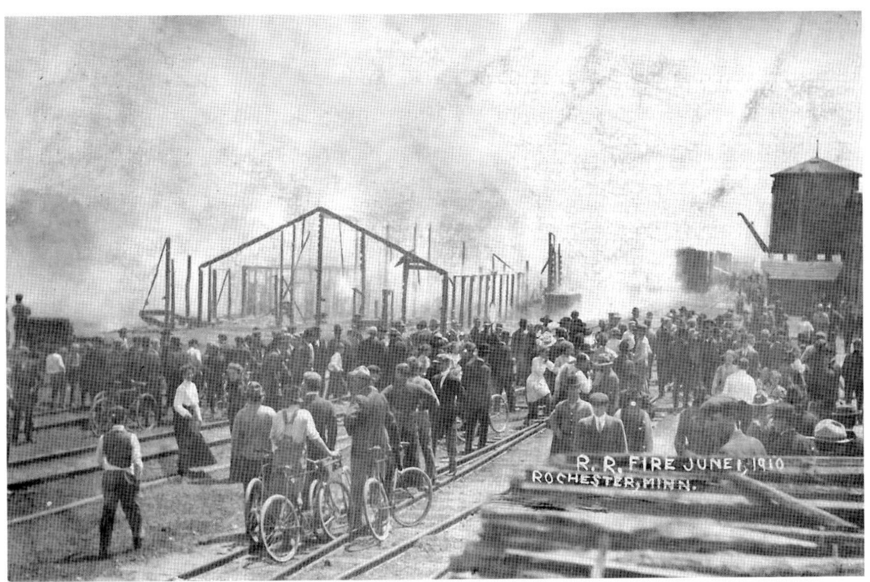

Postcard of C&GW train yard fire, June 1, 1910.

HORTON BLOCK FIRE
AT 1:30 A.M. JAN. 12th 1917
STEARNS
PHOTO

Postcard of Horton Block fire, January 12, 1917.

Rochester's Miracle Mile was constructed in 1952 and was the first strip mall in the city. It had twenty-six stores with two hundred thousand square feet of retail space and abundant parking. The anchor stores were Donaldson's department store at the north end, Snyder's Drugs at the south end and Red Owl grocery in the center. On February 21, 1971, a fire wiped out the south end, closing half of the stores. It was the largest and most costly fire in Rochester history. It was subsequently blamed on faulty furnace installation and improper storage of flammable materials at the hardware store.[74]

On July 18, 1979, fire broke out at Nelson Tire Town, a recapping facility at 4410 Nineteenth Street Northwest. Dense, billowing smoke filled the sky, visible twenty-five miles away. The burning pile contained over 225,000 tires. The remains in a deep pit continued to smolder for over a year. The loss was estimated at over $2 million, the costliest fire in city history.[75]

Other fires that are remembered because of historical images (postcards and newspaper photos) include the train depot fire on June 1, 1910; the Central School fire on September 1, 1910; the Baptist church fire on March 1, 1912; the Chicago and Northwestern train depot fire on October 25, 1914; the Masonic Temple fire on January 17, 1916; and the Horton Block fire on January 11–12, 1917.[76]

ROCHESTER PUBLIC LIBRARY

The Rochester Library Association was organized in 1865, with J.D. Blake as president; $1,000 was raised for the purchase of books, half from Blake. W.W. Mayo was a contributing founder. They sponsored annual visiting lecturers, including publisher and orator Horace Greeley, Black abolitionist Frederick Douglass and suffragette Anna E. Dickinson. In 1885, the city council began to support the library, and the library board became a city entity, with Bert W. Eaton appointed as president. In 1895, Colonel George Healy proposed to make a substantial donation ($5,000) to the library with a proviso that he, "being a free thinker, made a condition of his gift that there should be liberality in the choice of books purchased as the result of his bounty." Healy declared:

> *I desire that the library shall also contain books and reading matter of a liberal nature for the benefit of those who may desire to use them.... This*

> *donation is made upon these conditions. First, that no library work or book of any kind shall be barred or excluded from the Public Library of the city of Rochester by reason of its religious teachings, doctrines or views, if such books are not immoral....It is my desire that as a part of the books to be purchased by your board with the money which shall be donated by me, there shall be included the works of Thomas Paine, Robert G. Ingersoll and works of a similar nature.*

This proposal generated great controversy and was approved by the library board with a single vote majority. Leonard commented, "The money was paid over to the board and the community, apparently, does not care what kind of books are in the Library if only there are plenty of novels."

Prompted by a bequest of $5,000 from Huber Bastian in 1892, the city built the first public library building at the southwest corner of Zumbro and Main Street (First Avenue and Second Street Southwest). Dedicated in 1898 and built for a total cost of $15,000, it was an attractive two-story brick structure with a capacity of ten thousand volumes. It served the city until the construction of the second library building two blocks west on Second Street (see description under "Depression"). That building now houses Mayo Clinic Alix School of Medicine. The third public library building was at the

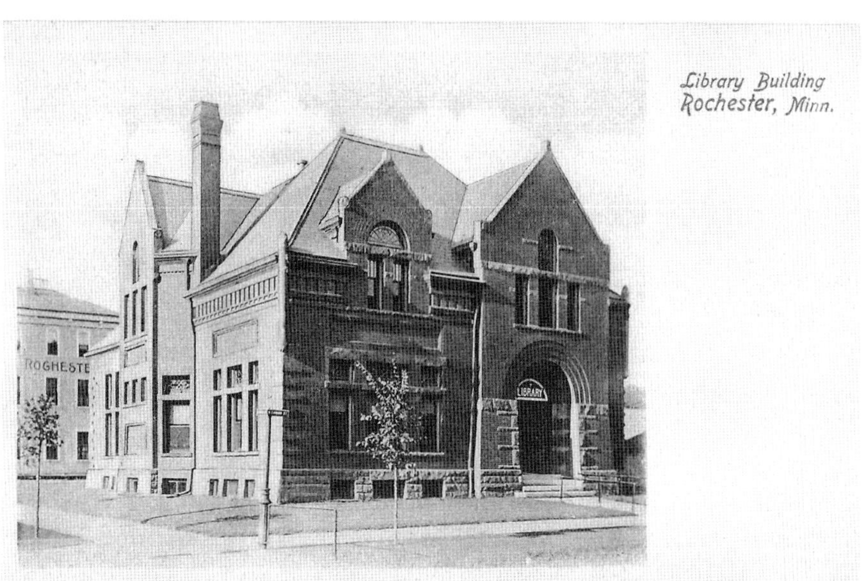

Postcard of original Rochester Public Library.

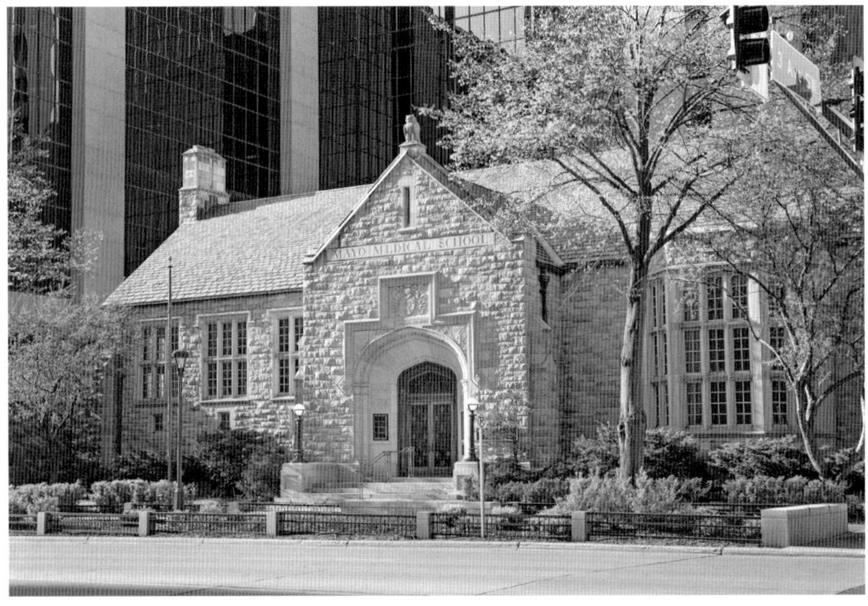

The second Rochester Public Library (now the Mitchell Student Center of the Mayo Clinic Alix School of Medicine). *Courtesy of Dean Riggott Photography.*

northeast corner of Broadway and First Street South, which was previously a JC Penny store. The current library is at Second Street and Civic Center Drive Southeast.[77]

MAYO GIFTS

The original layout of Rochester had only two parks: Central Park, on the block east of Charter House, marked as "Town Square" on the 1874 map of the city, and Cascade Park on Second Avenue and Eighth Street Northwest, which has always been called Goose Egg Park. In the days before parkland dedication became part of the city's land development process, there was no formal mechanism for the creation of new parks.

The Mayos knew the value of parks and cultural amenities and provided amply for them. They funded the salary of a band director for the school system. Along with hotelman John Cook, they donated money to purchase sixteen acres of land for Mayo Park in 1906. It was developed with bathhouses, walkways and bridges that were destroyed in the flood of June 23, 1908.

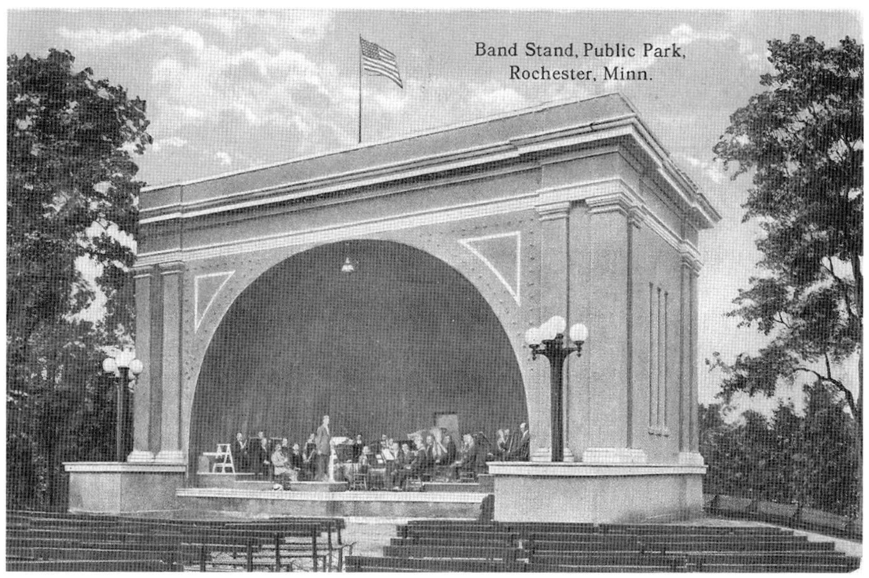

Postcard of Mayo Park bandshell.

The Mayos also donated two city blocks for College Park in 1906. It was so named because of its location at the top of College Street hill. It is now called St. Marys Park.[78] The park covered the very steep grade up Ninth Avenue from Second Street to Fourth Street Southwest, with a massive staircase set half the width of the block west of Ninth Avenue. Its uppermost portion can still be seen above the sandstone walls overlooking parking lots on Second Street.

The Mayos also donated the land for Mayo Field Ballpark in 1910. They funded a large bandshell built in Mayo Park for summertime concerts in 1915, and they paid the salary of the band director, Ralph L. Blakely.[79]

Their final gift to the city was Mayo Civic Auditorium, a $350,000 gift from Dr. Charlie and Mayo Properties Association, dedicated in the year both brothers died. Both were present for the groundbreaking on July 28, 1938. Both were on winter holiday in Tucson with their wives for the grand opening on March 8, 1939. They participated in the ceremony by a special two-way radio transmission. It included a 3,000-seat auditorium/hockey arena, a 1,200-seat theater and a ballroom. Later additions included a 7,200-seat sports/concert arena, a 25,000-square-foot exhibit hall, connections to the Civic Theater and the Art Center and, in 2017, a two-level convention

Victory Arch in City Park, Rochester, Minn.

MAYO PARK LOOKING EAST,
ROCHESTER, MINN.

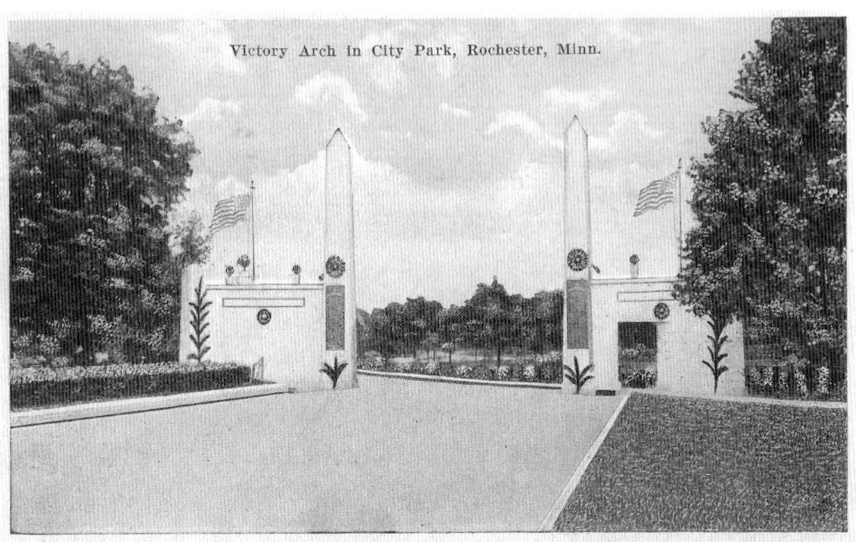

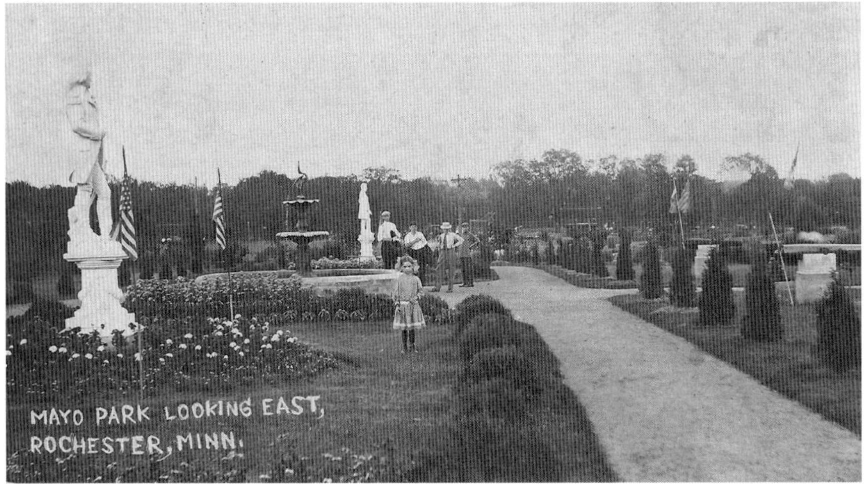

Top: Postcard of Victory Arches.

Bottom: Postcard of Washington and Lincoln statues.

center with a 40,000-square-foot three-section ballroom, sixteen meeting rooms and two boardrooms.[80]

Mayo Park has at times included a greenhouse, a sundial dedicated to honor the Daughters of the American Revolution and a zoo with a variety of North American mammals, including bear, bison, elk, wolves, foxes and other local species. A Native American totem pole from near Vancouver,

British Columbia (by the Nuu-chah-nulth or Nootka people), was placed in Mayo Park in 1932. It was last located by the old Rochester Art Center. It has been stored by the Park Department for years but is too fragile to place outdoors again.

A park mystery is the location and disposition of the Victory Arches, erected as a memorial to Olmsted County soldiers who died in World War I. Alan Calavano placed them at the entrance to the Statuary Park, coming off Second Street between First and Second Avenues Southeast. No one knows why they were taken down or what happened to them.

Another mystery is the disposition of the white Italian marble statues of Washington and Lincoln that were donated by the Mayos to the city. They were in the Statuary Park near the statue of W.W. Mayo. They were vandalized in 1938 and placed in storage. It is said that they were buried in a ravine in Soldier's Field in the 1950s near the YM/YWCA building. Their exact location is unknown.[81]

Revival—Billy Sunday, 1906

In 1906, for a month beginning in mid-January, Rochester hosted Reverend William A. "Billy" Sunday, a famous revivalist minister. He was a former professional baseball player for the Chicago Cubs, known for animated fundamentalist preaching with a colloquial style. He and his six staff members were welcomed by six Protestant churches and their ministers, who suspended their congregational activities for a month in deference to the revival. A tabernacle, seating 2,000, was built north of Center Street on First Avenue Northwest. The choirs of the congregations were combined into a super-choir. The revival meetings were held nearly every night and most afternoons throughout the month, with overflowing crowds. Collections went first to pay for the tabernacle and scheduled expenses and later to Reverend Sunday. A total of 1,296 individuals pledged as "converts."

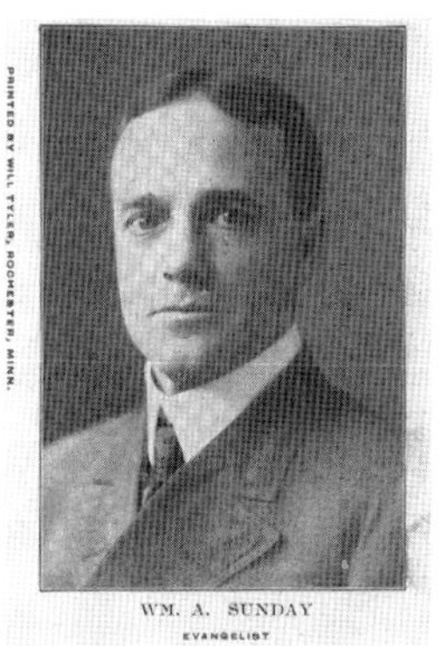

Postcard image of Reverend Billy Sunday.

At the conclusion of the revival, an effort was made to harness the enthusiasm in support of the Young Men's Christian Association. It succeeded, and contributions over $20,000 were made toward the $30,000 cost of a new building for the YMCA. It was built on Zumbro Street (Second Street Southwest), one lot west of Main Street (First Avenue Southwest), and served for over fifty years.[82]

Billy Sunday became an enthusiastic proponent of Mayo Clinic. He and his wife were both Mayo Clinic patients and were friends and correspondents of the Mayos for many years thereafter.

Women at Mayo Clinic—Great Beginnings with an Unfortunate Middle Act

William Worrall Mayo, the father of Drs. William J. and Charles H. Mayo, advocated for the inclusion of women in the practice of medicine. In the 1870s, he had a close collegial relationship with Dr. Harriet Preston, who maintained a practice of obstetrics and medical gynecology in Rochester. She referred her surgical patients to W.W. Mayo. Dr. Mayo proposed her for membership in the Minnesota State Medical Society in 1870 but was rebuked because women were not included as members. He persisted in his advocacy, despite a credible threat to his own licensure for collaborating with Dr. Preston. In 1880, the society reversed its position and admitted her to membership.[83] Dr. Mayo had a similar professional relationship with Dr. Ida Clarke.

W.W. Mayo's wife, Louise, was actively involved in his practice as his de facto business manager. She often advised patients on a variety of medical issues when he was absent on house calls or educational travel.

The partnership of W.W. Mayo with Mother Alfred Moes and the Sisters of St. Francis in establishing St. Marys Hospital was remarkable in many regards. Their association was criticized, more for the fact that the sisters were Catholic (he was Episcopalian) than that they were women. The sisters provided not only the money and the will to build St. Marys Hospital but also the nursing staff during its early history. Note that the Mayo surgical practice existed primarily at St. Marys for twenty-five years (1889–1914) before the first Mayo Clinic building was built.

The senior Mayo's inclusive attitude toward women was not missed by the Mayo brothers. As their practice grew in the late 1890s, they first recruited Drs. Augustus Stinchfield and Charlie's brother-in-law, Christopher Graham. Their next recruit, in 1898, was Dr. Gertrude Booker (later

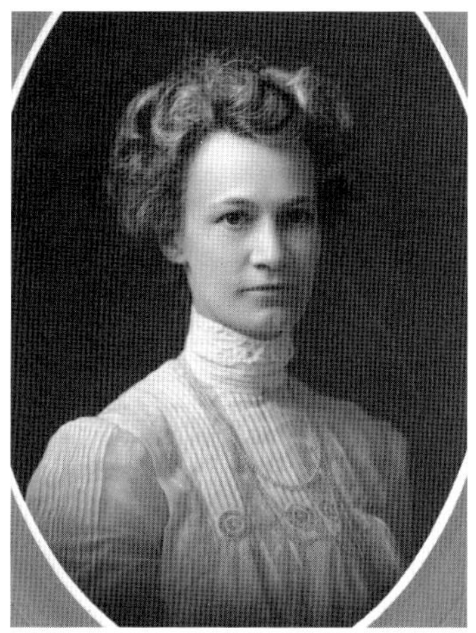

Dr. Gertrude Booker Granger.
By permission of Mayo Foundation for Medical Education and Research.

Granger), who practiced with Dr. Charlie managing medical aspects of ear, nose and throat and ophthalmology patients in their joint practice. She later succeeded Dr. Charlie as public health director for Rochester and Olmsted County. In 1899, the Mayos hired Dr. Isabella Herb, whose practice included anesthesia and pathology. She left in 1904 and moved to Chicago. In 1908, Dr. Leda Stacy was recruited to the practice, becoming the third female physician in the association (the second out of eleven active physicians at that point), at a time when there were very few women in American medicine. The Mayos included other women as key members of their organization, including Edith Graham (later Mayo) as their original nurse anesthetist and nurse educator; Maud Mellish (later Wilson) as director of publications, the medical library and medical illustrations; and Mabel Root as manager of medical records. Women have always made up a large majority of Mayo Clinic employees, particularly allied health staff (clerical, technical, administrative, et cetera) and nurses.[84]

Mayo Clinic continued to train and recruit women (physicians and others) throughout the careers of the Mayo brothers; however after they retired and throughout the Great Depression, nearly all of the women members of the physician staff left Rochester. (Some were dismissed; others, for example Leda Stacy, left after their practice was undermined by the loss of women colleagues.) No women were hired to the consultant staff between 1935 and 1948.[85] During those years, and for many years after, it was standard practice that if a physician couple was recruited, the husband would be recruited and the wife, if she wished to continue medical practice, would join the staff of Olmsted Medical Group (OMG). If a physician pair married, the wife was expected to resign from the staff either to practice at OMG or to give up medicine. The vast predominance of male physicians did not begin to change until the establishment of Mayo Medical School in 1972, with associated federal mandates for inclusion of women leading to more women in training programs. Even then the number of women recruited to the staff and higher roles of physician leadership grew very slowly until the mid- to late 1990s and after 2000. Many of the most senior women currently on the consultant staff (attending physicians) or recent emerita had difficulties in their paths to joining the staff, which would not be likely to occur today. Progress has been made in recent decades. The Mayo Clinic staff is now a better, though still improving, reflection of our culture. Women have long since achieved or surpassed parity in admissions to the medical school and most residencies and have made substantial inroads in appointments to the staff, productivity and recognition in research and education and assignment to many of the highest administrative and leadership positions. Recently, it was shown that Mayo Clinic with a "structured compensation model" achieves gender equality in salaries for most employees, with the two remaining exceptions due to historic dominance of men in leadership positions and overrepresentation of men in highly compensated specialties.[86] Efforts continue to recruit women to leadership positions and to historically male-dominated specialties.

DR. LEDA STACY, A PIONEER IN FOUR MEDICAL FIELDS, 1908

When Leda June Stacy first joined the Mayo practice in 1908, she worked as a physician anesthetist. In 1910, she was asked to join Dr. Graham in the internal medicine practice supporting the Mayos' surgical practice. In 1915, Dr. Will asked her to develop the new practice of radium therapy (later called therapeutic radiology and eventually radiation oncology). She traveled to Baltimore to learn the new medical practice at Johns Hopkins Hospital. After training, she returned to Rochester carrying a supply of radium in her luggage! After she started the practice and chaired the Section on Radium Therapy, she was asked, in 1917, to establish a section of medical gynecology. Thus, she was a pioneer in four different specialties. After twenty-eight years, she left Mayo Clinic in 1935 to move to White Plains, New York, where she lived with her friend

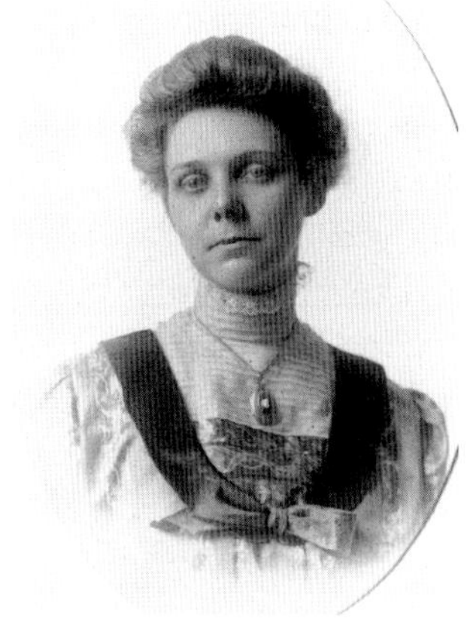

Dr. Leda Stacy. *By permission of Mayo Foundation for Medical Education and Research.*

and former Mayo colleague Dr. L. Mary Moench. Dr. Stacy practiced in the controversial field of family planning until her retirement in 1966 at the age of eighty-three. She died in 1973 at the age of ninety and is buried at Oakwood Cemetery in her family plot next to the Mayo family plot. She is one of my professional heroes. One of the six "Firms" to which internal medicine residents are assigned is named in her honor.[87]

Mayowood, 1911

The Mayo brothers and their families were neighbors in similar wood-frame houses on College Street (Fourth Street) from early in their careers until 1911–12. They shared a summer cottage at a millpond called Lake Allis (later called Lake Shady) near Oronoco and shared ownership of the first of Dr. Will's three riverboats, the *Oronoco*. (The next was the *Minnesota* followed by the *North Star*.) However, both Dr. Charlie and Edith believed they and their children would be better off if they actually lived in the country on a real working farm. They bought property on the Zumbro, three miles southwest of town.

They gave their "red house" to the local YMCA, and it served for many years as headquarters for the YWCA and then as housing for single women. It was torn down in the dead of night in 1986 without a permit, environmental impact assessment or historical assessment under direction of a local realtor, who paid a trivial fine for lack of permits and sold the cleared property to Mayo Clinic for a parking lot.

The "Big House" at Mayowood was designed by Dr. Charlie. (It is uncertain whether he had the help of an architectural firm.) It has thirty-eight rooms, sufficient to accommodate Charlie and Edith's eight children (six biological and two adopted), plus many visitors. They began with 320 acres but continued to acquire adjacent farms, eventually owning 3,000 acres with seven functional farms, as well as greenhouses, a horse track, game preserves and multiple outbuildings of various kinds. A lake was formed by a hydroelectric dam on the South Fork of the Zumbro River. It had multiple islands, a Japanese teahouse, extensive gardens and a Venetian gondola.

Dr. Charlie recognized raw milk as a source of tuberculosis. He advocated for pasteurization of milk. He led a successful, though highly contentious, campaign to mandate pasteurization in the city. After that campaign,

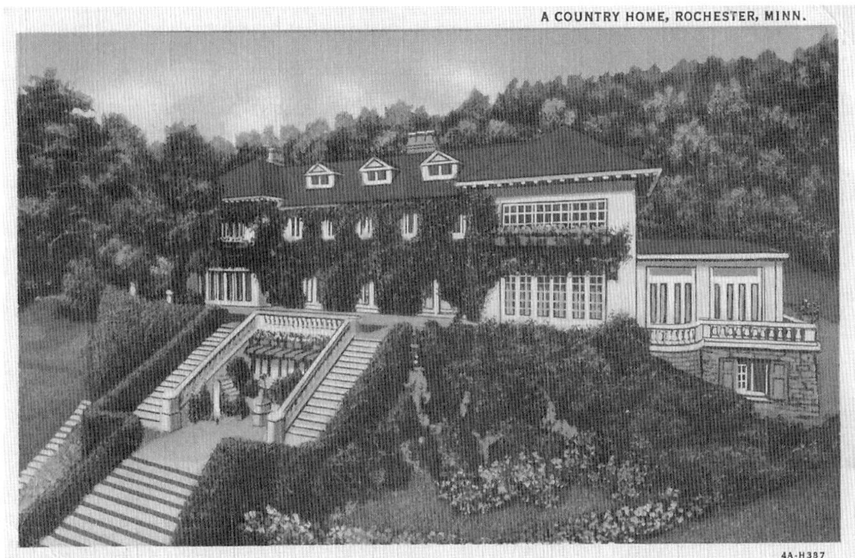

Postcard of Mayowood.

in 1912, Dr. Charlie was appointed public health officer for the City of Rochester. He introduced scientific methods into the practice of public health locally. He also organized garbage collection for the city. Prior to that, most households in the city dumped their garbage in backyards and alleys. He established a hog feeding facility to process food waste garbage. It maintained scrupulous standards for infection control and proved to be highly profitable.[88]

After Dr. Charlie died in 1939, Edith moved to Ivy Lodge at Mayowood, and their son Dr. Charles William "Chuck" Mayo and his wife, Alice, moved into the Big House with their eight children. Over the years, many dignitaries visited the house, including President Franklin Delano Roosevelt and Eleanor Roosevelt, Helen Keller, Adlai Stevenson, the king of Nepal and King Faisal of Saudi Arabia. In 1965, to ensure the house's historic preservation, Dr. Chuck and Alice and their children presented Mayowood and some of its surrounding acreage to the Olmsted County Historical Society. In 1967, it was declared a Minnesota Historic Site, and in 1970, it was named to the National Register of Historic Places. The Olmsted Historical Society and the Friends of Mayowood struggled for years to maintain the enormous house, but it deteriorated. In 2013, Mayo Clinic assumed ownership and now maintains the house. Mayo Clinic has spent millions of dollars repairing the aging structure, including rebuilding a major portion of the foundation and bringing the facilities up to contemporary standards for heating and air conditioning, technology and accessibility. The house is open to the public throughout the year, with regularly scheduled tours. The History Center retained rights to use the house part of the time.

The First Mayo Clinic: The Medical Block, the Red Brick Building, the 1914 Building

Outpatient clinical facilities of Mayo Clinic evolved over many years. W.W. Mayo had his office on Third Street Southwest. When Dr. Will joined him in his practice in 1883, they moved their offices to a larger space on the upper level of the Cook Block, also known as the Massey's Building, at the southeast corner of Second Street and First Avenue Southwest. That site sufficed until 1901, when they moved to still larger quarters in the new Masonic Temple at the northwest corner of the same intersection. Over the next decade, the offices in the Masonic Temple grew both in space and complexity, including connected spaces in adjacent buildings.

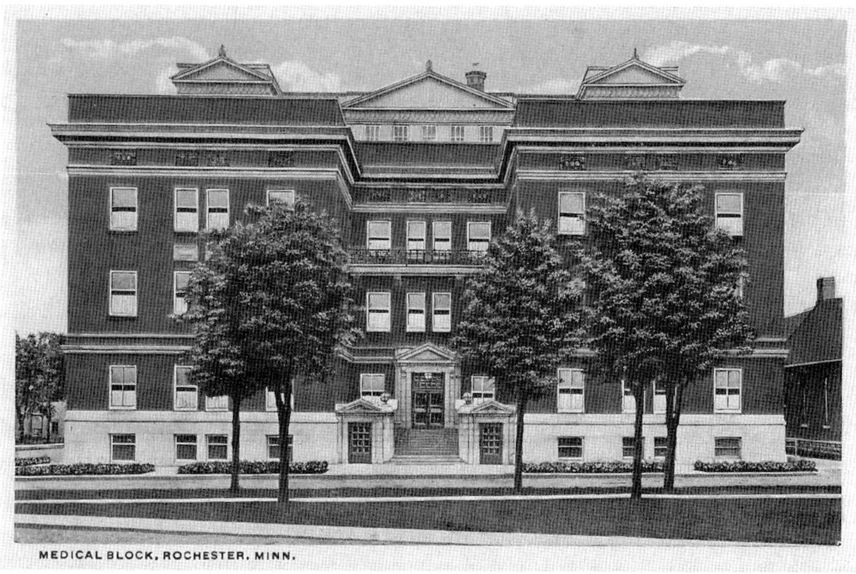

Postcard of original Mayo Clinic—the Medical Block, the Red Brick building, the 1914 Building.

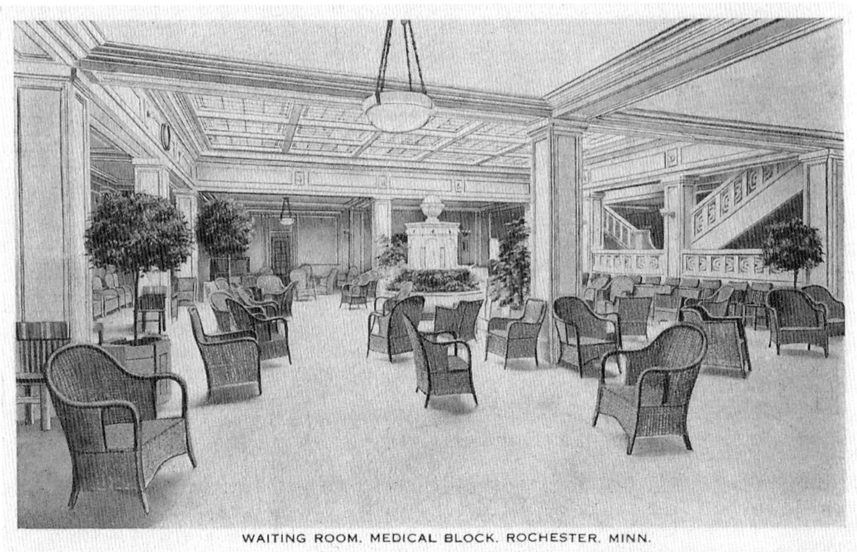
WAITING ROOM. MEDICAL BLOCK. ROCHESTER. MINN.

Postcard of the interior of 1914 Building.

A library annex was constructed behind the building to the west. The practice became more and more crowded, prompting experiments with split work shifts. Finally, in 1912, Dr. Henry Plummer's longstanding recommendation to construct a new facility was approved, and he was appointed to chair a building committee that included business manager Harry Harwick and laboratory director Dr. Louis Wilson. Plummer spoke the next morning with Franklin Ellerbe of the Ellerbe and Rounds architectural firm. Dr. Plummer knew of their work from their recently completed Zumbro Hotel, designed for hotelier John Kahler and built by the local contractor Garfield Schwartz.

Dr. Plummer provided strong leadership with the concept of building workspaces to serve work groups of the evolving medical specialties. The design of the building was developed after Dr. Plummer and colleagues conferred with each of the specialty groups to determine how they needed to work within their group and in collaboration with others. From that anticipated workflow, Dr. Plummer and the architects designed the building to facilitate the organization, essentially designing what became known as multispecialty group practice and building a facility to support it. They developed a standard generic Mayo Clinic examination room and layout that remains the Mayo Clinic standard to the present. The design process included organized and coordinated approaches to traffic flow, medical records, appointments, data recording and reporting, X-ray handling and storage and a multitude of other processes that ultimately contributed to the organization and practice of Mayo Clinic.

A cornerstone was laid on October 9, 1912. Dr. Will stated, "Within its walls all classes of people, the poor as well as the rich, without regard to color or creed, shall be cared for without discrimination."

Dr. Plummer also had a strong aesthetic intent. Dr. Leda Stacy, a pioneering early member of the Mayo firm, described it in her memoir:

> *I remember when the 1914 building was complete. Dr. Will was rather disturbed, fearing it was too big and too elegant. Dr. Henry S. Plummer, however, had deliberately included a degree of distinction in the plans of the building. He thought it ought to be beautiful in its exterior and interior aspects, for he felt that perhaps in many instances the patients and their relatives would be surrounded by architectural beauty for the first time and would thus be helped to find some measure of peace and solace while waiting their appointments with the physician.*[89]

The exterior was a Greek Revival design with dark red Pennsylvania brick and cream-colored Missouri stone trim. The lobby was beautifully arranged with over three hundred large comfortable wicker chairs and architectural accents including Rookwood tile fixtures and Tiffany glass skylights. The 1914 Building established the concept, followed with all subsequent Mayo Clinic buildings, which is sometimes called the "Healing Environment" of Mayo Clinic. (See "Art and Healing," pages 180–185).

The new building had a lintel over the main entrance with the words "Mayo Clinic," the first time the term was applied to a building. Prior to that, visiting physicians had used the term "Mayo's clinics" to describe the teaching sessions the Mayos held for visiting clinicians to demonstrate surgical techniques and other clinical skills. Note that this was thirty-one years after Dr. Will Mayo joined his father's medical practice and long after the Mayo brothers were world renowned as surgeons.

The facility was built on the site of the original Mayo family home on the southeast corner of Second Avenue and First Street Southwest, across from Central School. It stood there for seventy-two years, until it was demolished to make way for the Siebens Building, despite its designation in the National Register of Historic Places. Part of the rationale for demolishing it was a concern about its structural integrity; however, it took three weeks with a wrecking ball to knock it down. It was difficult to demolish without damaging the Plummer Building and so-called Connecting Link. If you look at the Plummer Building now, you will notice the entryway is a distinct three-story structure attached to the north side of the Plummer Building, connecting it to the south side of the Siebens Building. It once linked the Plummer to the 1914 Building, while the interiors functioned as connected spaces at levels one through three.[90]

The Foundation House, Residence of Dr. Will and Hattie Mayo, 1915

Not long after Dr. Charlie and Edith moved into Mayowood, Dr. Will and Hattie started planning their mansion at 701 Fourth Street Southwest (College Street) on a high point of the city. The lot was previously occupied by the home of city founder George Head. According to Clapesattle, Dr. Will took relatively little role in the design of the house. "Dr. Will asked only that it have a tower like the one from which he had watched the stars with his mother." He wanted a home that would allow him to entertain large numbers of visiting physicians and scientists. Franklin Ellerbe was the principal architect. His son, Thomas Ellerbe, described it as "a gracious Tudor home with spacious grounds and gardens, which became a social center for the community and its important visitors." Its style is also described as Renaissance Revival.

It was built with Kasota limestone (quarried near the town of Kasota between Mankato and St. Peter). It contains twenty-four thousand square feet in forty-seven rooms with many meeting/dining rooms. It has an organ for entertainment and a third-floor ballroom for social occasions. The five-story observation tower looks out over the city and includes a private study for Dr. Will and a billiard table. Dr. Will and Hattie planned from the beginning to leave the house, later in their lives, to the clinic for meetings and promotion of the functions of the clinic, particularly education. They transferred ownership in 1938. Today, the house is commonly known as the Foundation House. The grounds are beautifully maintained in a park-like setting. The Foundation House is used for private Mayo Clinic functions and is not open to the public. It is well regarded for hospitable staff and excellent cuisine. A special treat frequently served at the start of the meal is popovers with strawberry preserves. Service is always impeccable. Before Mayo Clinic became

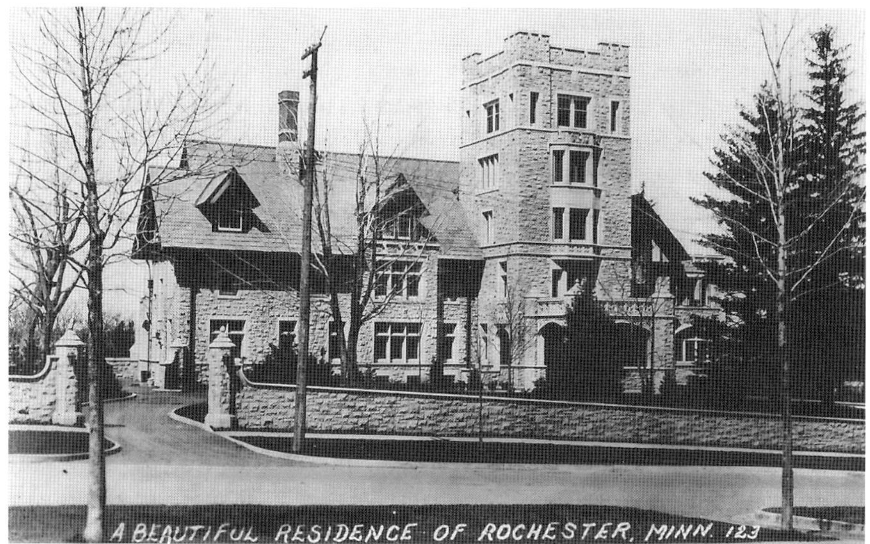

Postcard of the Foundation House, the residence of Dr. Will and Hattie Mayo.

smoke-free in 1986, the Foundation House served cigars after meals. While President Lyndon Johnson served on the Board of Trustees, the former no-alcohol policy at the Foundation House, established by Dr. Will, was changed to permit Johnson to have his glass of bourbon in the evening. Since then, wine has been commonly served with meals.

Dr. Will's library on the first floor still houses his book collection. He was a fan of popular literature, particularly westerns. He graded his books with a letter grade, *A–F*, and kept only books he graded *C* or better. The house contains several lamps by Louis Comfort Tiffany, featuring beautiful stained-glass shades. Several belonged to Dr. Will and Hattie. Others are from the estate of Barbara Woodward Lips. Other decorative elements include Western art, including bronze sculptures by Frederick Remington and an original watercolor by Charles Russell, who was a patient of Dr. Will.

The newel post at the lower end of the main staircase is central in the entry area. It has a hollow at its upper end covered by a wooden cap. The Mayos kept small change there for deliveries, and the tradition has been continued with foreign guests leaving foreign currency in the recessed space. The house is listed in the U.S. National Register of Historic Places.

Boats—*Oronoco*, *Minnesota*, *North Star*

Of the Mayo brothers, Dr. Will was the sailor. Dr. Charlie was co-owner of their first boat, the *Oronoco*, but whereas Dr. Will loved traveling on the river, Dr. Charlie was less enamored. Regarding cars and boats, Dr. Will said, "I can rest if what I'm sitting in is moving." Dr. Charlie would often disappear when the boat was docked to engage in conversation with locals. After the *Oronoco*, Dr. Charlie's interests focused on his farm. The Mayos were extremely generous in their entertainment on the boats, often hosting large parties for weekend or longer outings. They included not only physician staff but also allied health staff, including Sisters of St. Francis. The Mayo brothers and their captain and crew ran a tight ship. They always insisted that during the boating season the crew and boat be ready to cast off with ten minutes notice.

The *Oronoco* was acquired by the brothers when a lumber firm they invested in failed in 1913. As part of the liquidation of assets, they acquired a riverboat called the *John H. Rich*. They had it refitted as a pleasure craft and renamed it the *Oronoco* (after the town, not the river, which is spelled *Orinoco*). It was 132.0 feet long, 30.5 feet abeam and had a 4.7-foot draft. They sold it in 1917. It was subsequently owned by a coal company, was renamed the *Ben Franklin* after the company and worked as a towboat until it was destroyed by fire in Cincinnati in 1935.

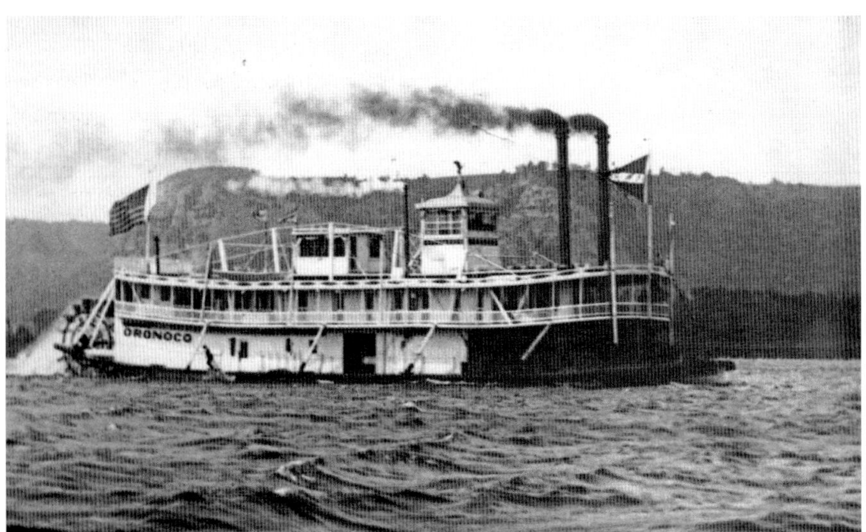

The *Oronoco*. *By permission of Mayo Foundation for Medical Education and Research.*

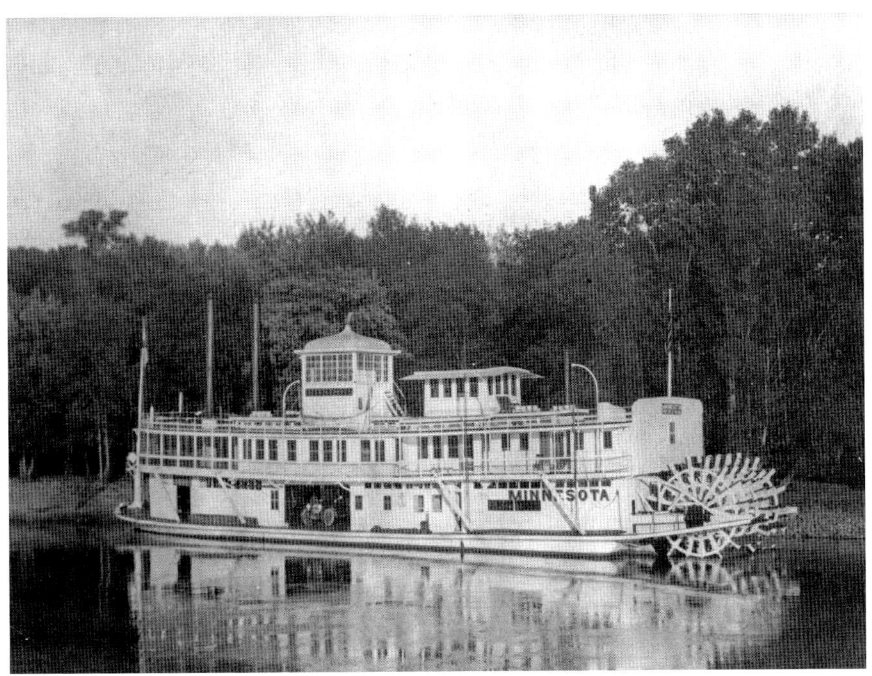

The *Minnesota. By permission of Mayo Foundation for Medical Education and Research.*

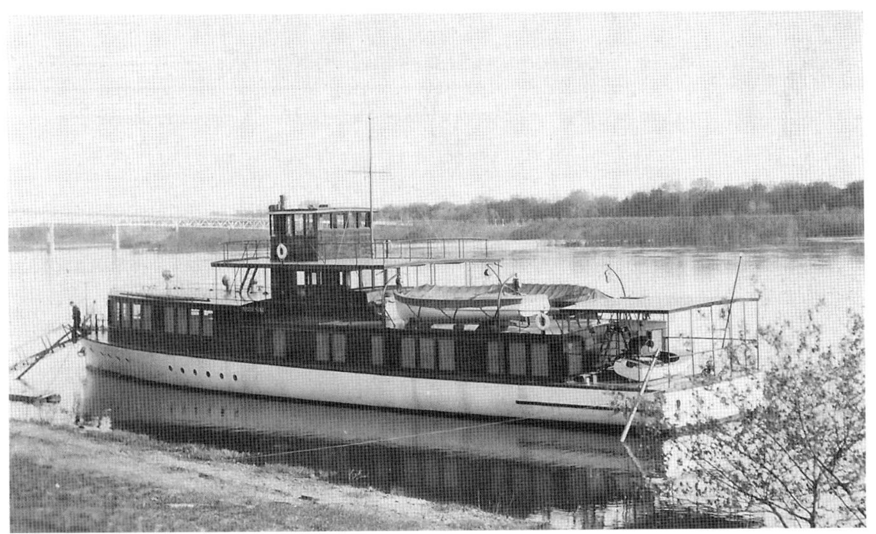

Postcard of the *North Star.*

The next boat was built for the Mayos and was completed in 1916. Named the *Minnesota*, it was a steam-powered sternwheeler, 115.0 feet long, 30.0 feet abeam, 5.2-foot draft, with a 180-horsepower engine capable of ten miles per hour. It had a unique three-pitch whistle. On the top level behind the captain's wheelhouse stood a second house for Dr. Will's study. Those two features made it recognizable from miles away. It carried automobiles on board for local travel or overland return home if needed. It was sold in 1922 and renamed the *General Allen*. It deteriorated until it was restored in 1966 and outfitted as a floating restaurant. It was destroyed by fire in the 1970s.

The last boat was the *North Star*, built in 1922. It had twin 250-horsepower, 8-cylinder gasoline engines and twin propeller drive. It was 120.0 feet long and 22.0 feet abeam with 3.5-foot draft. It would sleep twenty-five and cruised at twelve miles per hour with a maximum speed of fourteen miles per hour. It also carried an automobile for shore excursions. They entertained on it extensively and took many trips downriver and along the inland waterway on the Atlantic Coast. After 1932, during the Depression, traveling in such luxury seemed inappropriate to Dr. Will, so they took no more long trips. It was sold in 1938, with the proceeds given to the section of social work to benefit the indigent. It was subsequently used as a training vessel by the U.S. Army.[91]

THE NATIONAL GUARD ARMORY, "THE CASTLE," 1916

The distinctive former National Guard Armory, now called the Castle, sits at the southwest corner of the intersection of North Broadway and Second Street. The three-story brick Romanesque Revival building is distinctive for its octagonal tower and crenellated roofline. It was designed to house the Minnesota National Guard's Rochester Machine Gun Company Third Infantry as directed by the Militia Act of 1903. It was built on land purchased by the state in 1915. The $39,000 cost was split between the city and the state. It was dedicated on February 10, 1916, at a gala event attended by seven hundred, followed by a dinner and dance in the drill hall, which could seat two thousand or accommodate a basketball game. It has been listed in the National Register of Historic Places since 1980. During World War I and World War II, the armory was used for military purposes. During peace times, it served as a community center, hosting concerts, dances, sporting events, high school graduations, political rallies, car shows and cooking demonstrations.

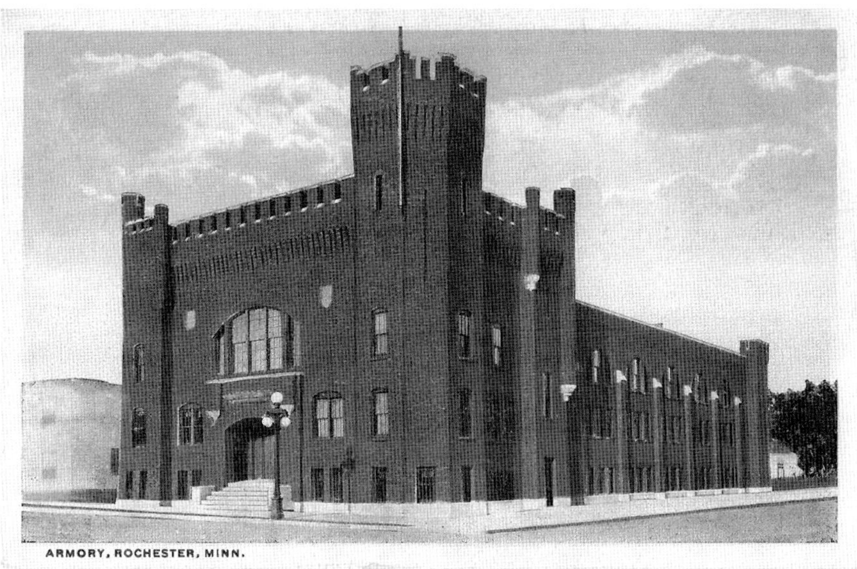

Postcard of the National Guard Armory.

The building's military use and state ownership ended in the 1970s. From 1979 to 2016, it housed the Rochester Senior Citizens Center. In September 2017, the city sold the building to a private for-profit group that repurposed the building's three levels, with a restaurant on the lowest level, commercial space and art exhibition on the middle level and a performance space on the upper level.[92]

Plummer House, 1917

In 1917, Dr. Henry Stanley Plummer and his wife, Daisy Berkman Plummer, began designing their home, which they called Quarry Hill. It later came to be known as the Plummer House of the Arts or just the Plummer House. Built in the remains of a quarry, the house and water tower are visible from a wide area because they are built on a high shoulder of land adjacent to the Rochester neighborhood called "Pill Hill" (so called because of the many Mayo Clinic doctors who live there). It was designed in Jacobethan Tudor Revival style by Thomas Ellerbe, son of Franklin Ellerbe, in conjunction with Dr. Plummer. Construction was completed in 1924. The exterior is stucco with limestone and wood trim and a slate roof; 25 percent of the limestone used for the exterior was quarried on site. The interior has forty-nine rooms, ten bathrooms, nine bedrooms, five fireplaces and a ballroom on the third floor. There are eleven thousand square feet of living space and over twenty thousand square feet total, including the basement and attached garage and greenhouse.

Dr. Plummer was an innovator both in clinical practice and in design. This was as true with his house as it was with the 1914 Building and the Plummer Building. Innovative features of the house, mostly designed by Dr. Plummer, include a central vacuum system, an intercom system, a security system, a dumbwaiter, electric and gas lighting, the first gas furnace in the city, garage door openers and many other special features.

The grounds, which were fashioned from a hilltop quarry, also include gardens, ponds, an underground sprinkler system, a gazebo, a heated pool and a distinctive grey stucco water tower that also has an observation room/study used by Dr. Plummer. Housing for the house manager is attached. The foundation of the greenhouse remains, awaiting funding for reconstruction. The footprint of the kidney-shaped pool is visible on the south side of the house, filled in as a garden. The heating system was replaced recently with the addition of air conditioning, which dramatically improved the house's preservation and usability.

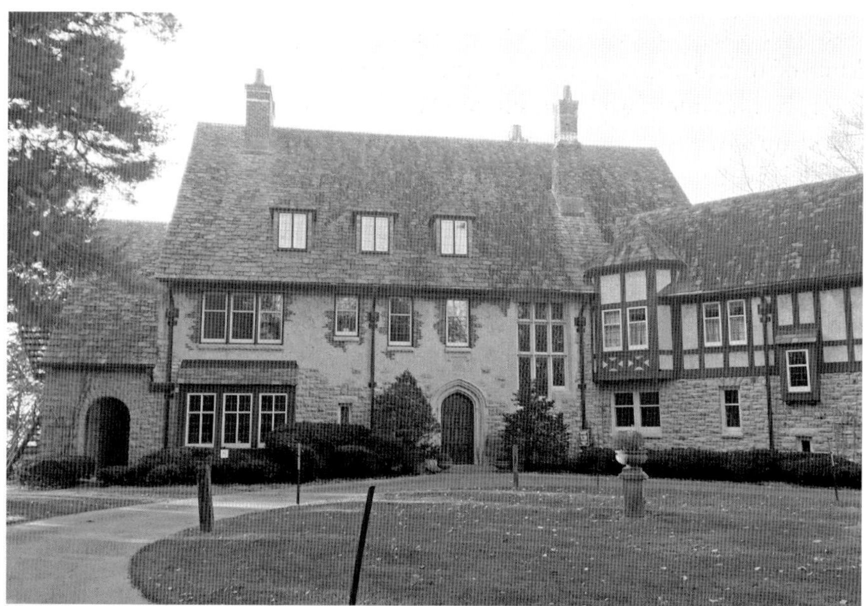

North elevation of the Plummer House on "Pill Hill."

Not accessible to the public is a system of tunnels underneath the house, dug into the underlying sandstone, that connects the house with the water tower. In addition, a 220-foot-long-by-18-foot-wide underground passageway connects the main house with what was the caretaker's house at the bottom of the hill.

When the house was built, the property totaled sixty-five acres. After Dr. Plummer died in 1936, Mrs. Plummer sold all but eleven acres. The sold property was developed as a new neighborhood, originally called Belmont Slope. It includes Tenth Street, Plummer Circle and Plummer Lane Southwest.

Daisy Plummer was a talented musician and patron of the arts in Rochester. She was the daughter of Gertrude Berkman (née Mayo), thus she was the niece of Drs. Will and Charlie. The Plummers had two adopted children, Robert and Gertrude. Dr. Plummer died of a stroke in 1936. Daisy Plummer and the family continued to live at the house until 1969. In her later years, although she became blind, she knew the house so well that she moved graciously through it and was able to give thorough tours to guests.

In 1969, she donated the house, designated the Plummer House of the Arts, to the Rochester Art Center for use and enjoyment by the residents of Rochester. Three years later, the house and eleven surrounding acres were turned over to the Rochester Parks and Recreation Department, with better resources for maintenance and management as part of the parks system. Most of the furniture currently in the house is original. Recent acquisitions from the Plummer family, mostly smaller artifacts originally from the house, are exhibited in cabinets and complement the furniture. Access to the grounds is free, and the house is open on a limited basis for tours. The house and grounds are a favorite venue for weddings and private social occasions, available by rental from the Rochester Parks and Recreation Department. The Plummer House was added to the National Register of Historic Places in 1975. Mrs. Plummer died in 1976.[93]

World War I, 1917–18

The United States entered the war on April 6, 1917. Rochester's Company D of the National Guard was called to active duty on September 7. The Axis Powers surrendered only fourteen months later on November 11, 1918, during the second and most severe peak of the great influenza pandemic.

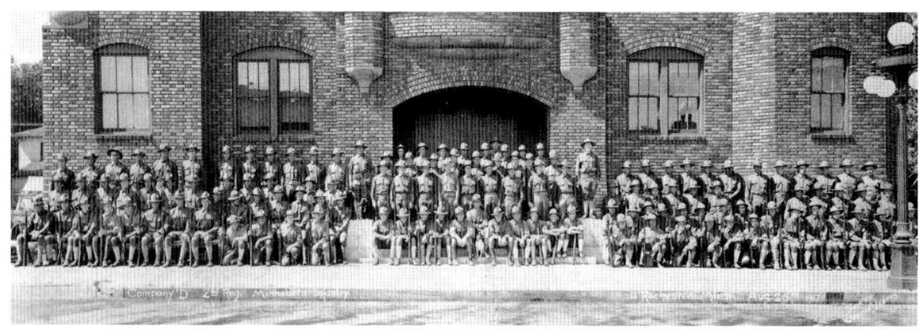

Panoramic of Company D. *Courtesy of the History Center of Olmsted County.*

In 1916, the Medical Board for National Defense (Dr. Will was chair and Dr. Charlie a member), working through the Red Cross, organized fifty base hospitals. Base Hospital 26 was organized by the University of Minnesota in cooperation with Mayo Clinic and with financial support and staff from Mayo Clinic. It was located near Dijon in east central France. It received patients from July 23, 1918. It was called the Mayo Unit and specialized in surgical care of battle casualties. They cared for 7,200 soldiers before returning home in May 1919.[94]

THE WAR IS ALMOST OVER! LET'S RENAME ALL THE STREETS BUT KEEP BROADWAY AND THIRD STREET THE SAME! 1918

On July 9, 1918, nearly all streets were renamed in Rochester, Minnesota, abandoning a set of names of persons, trees, flowers and other such memorable names. In the words of the *Post Bulletin*'s Answer Man:

> *When Rochester changed "Zumbro Street" to "Second Street Southwest," the city stripped away some of the beautifully descriptive and meaningful ways we understood our little world here. In 1918, the U.S. was at war, the old world was passing away and a new, post-war modernity was being born.... The world was changing quickly, and Rochester leaders thought it was time to streamline the names of streets and "modernize" the system. So, gone with the wind were street names that had been used since territorial days and soon after, such as Olmsted, Glencoe, State, College, Clark, Washington, Liberty and a virtual forest of trees names, including Oak and Elm.*[95]

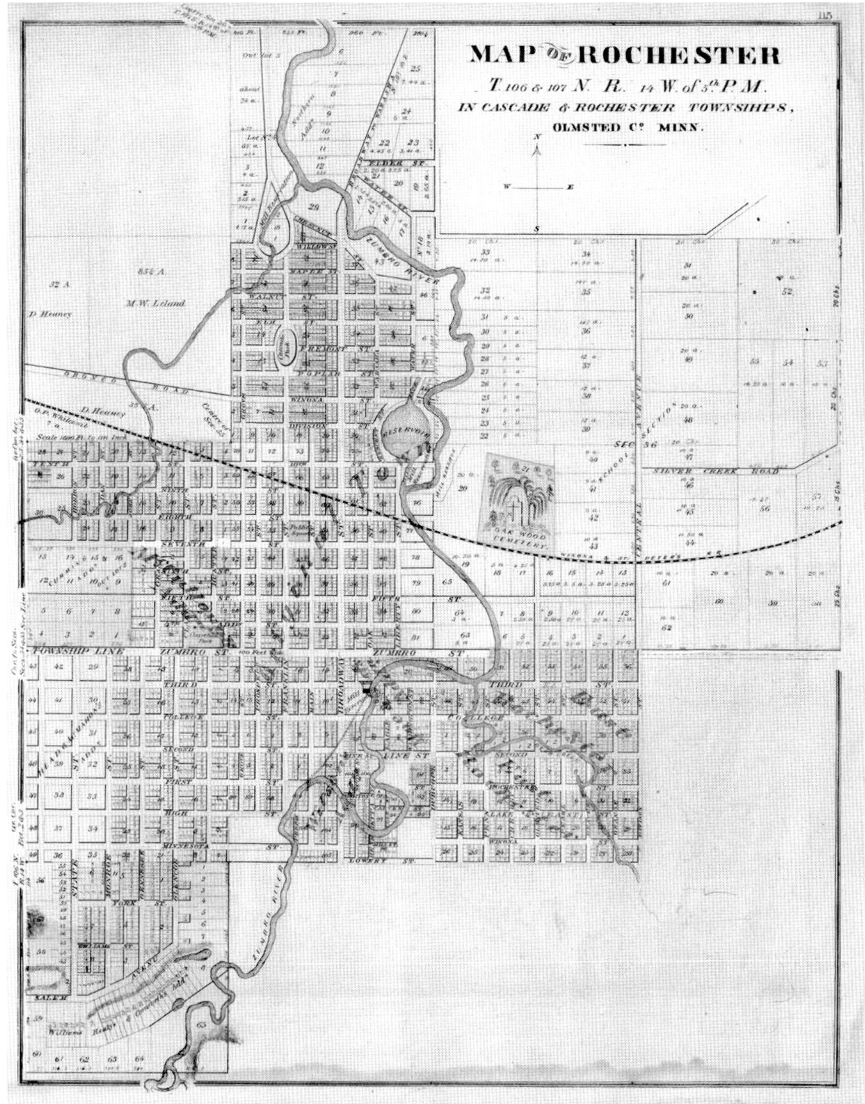

Map of Rochester. *From Andreas's* Historical Atlas of the State of Minnesota, *1874.*

The new system used Cartesian coordinates with four quadrants and axial dividing streets at Broadway and the former Fifth Street, now renamed Center Street. Streets are numbered in sequence as a function of distance from the center. North–south streets are called avenues and east–west streets are called streets. Andreas's 1874 *Historical Atlas of the State of Minnesota* includes a map of Rochester showing the historic street names.[96] Local history buffs have advocated for changing back a few of the historic downtown street names, particularly Zumbro (Second) and College (Fourth) Streets, but with little apparent impact.[97]

Table 1
A Sample of Street Names, New and Old

Seventh Street North	Winona Street (Oronoco Road)
Sixth Street North	Division Street
Fifth Street North	Tenth Street
Second Street North	Seventh Street
Center Street	Fifth Street
Second Street South	Zumbro Street
Third Street South	Third Street
Fourth Street South	College Street
Fifth Street South	Second Street
Sixth Street South	First Street
Seventh Street South	High Street
Eighth Street South	Minnesota Street
Ninth Street South	York Street
Ninth Avenue West	State Street
Eighth Avenue West	Monroe Street
Seventh Avenue West	Genesee Street (Grant Street)
Sixth Avenue West	Glencoe Street (Clark Street)
Fifth Avenue West	Hunter Street (Dacotah Street)

Fourth Avenue West	Grove Street
Third Avenue West	Prospect Street
Second Avenue West	Franklin Street
First Avenue West	Main Street
Broadway Avenue	Broadway Street
First Avenue Southeast	Oak Street
Second Avenue Southeast	Liberty Street
Third Avenue Southeast	Dubuque Street
Fourth Avenue Southeast	Kansas Street
Fifth Avenue Southeast	Penn Street
Sixth Avenue Southeast	Cherry Street
Seventh Avenue Southeast	Oakwood Street
Eighth Avenue Southeast	Pearl Street
Ninth Avenue Southeast	Beaver Street
Tenth Avenue Southeast	Orange Street
Eleventh Avenue Southeast	Central Street/Davidson Avenue

Influenza Pandemic, 1918

The "Spanish flu" of 1918–19 was an H1N1 influenza that originated in birds and was first spread by military personnel. The virus was thought to have arisen from animals in the American Midwest. The first reported human case was at Fort Riley, Kansas, on March 11, 1918. *Spanish* was a misnomer. Spain was a neutral country in the war and did not censor reports of the early outbreak, unlike combatant countries, giving the mistaken impression that it started and spread there. The actual 1918 virus has been re-created for research purposes from lung tissues of Alaskan Native influenza victims who were buried in permafrost.

The pandemic occurred in three waves, spanning more than a year from the spring of 1918 to the summer of 1919. The first wave was milder, with relatively few deaths. The second came in the fall of 1918 and was far more deadly. It subsided in the early winter until a smaller third wave in the late winter and spring of 1919, tapering off in summer. The illness was characterized by rapid onset, often in previously healthy persons, with a severe, often hemorrhagic, viral pneumonia or pulmonary edema. It could progress from initial mild symptoms to respiratory failure, cyanosis, hemorrhage and death in a matter of hours or very few days. Among those who survived the onset of the viral pneumonia, many died of secondary bacterial pneumonia after a few days. Mortality was highest among children under five years, young adults of twenty to forty years and the elderly. The high mortality in healthy young adults was an unusual and tragic feature of this pandemic.

When the earliest cases occurred in the spring of 1918, the Mayo brothers met with Sister Joseph to plan for the outbreak. The sisters purchased the Lincoln Hotel, next door to the east of St. Marys, and had it remodeled for use as the St. Marys Isolation Hospital. It opened in June and filled quickly in September when the second wave started. Extra cots were needed during the worst of the pandemic, but it served its purpose admirably. Staffing was difficult because numbers were already depleted by the war and then

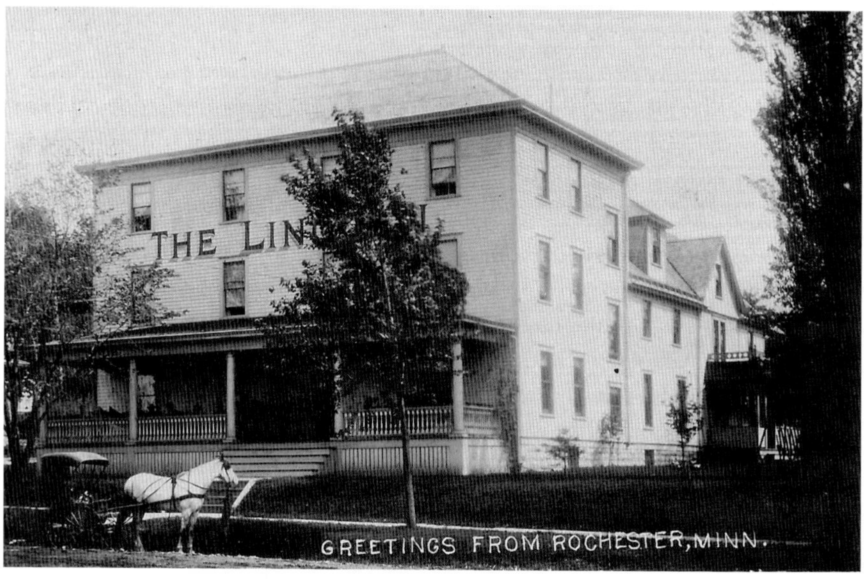

Postcard of the Lincoln, the Isolation Hospital of 1918.

many staff, including the Sisters of St. Francis, became ill from exposure to patients. The clinic and hospital reduced elective visits and surgical procedures. The workload forced the depleted staff to work longer hours and rely on community volunteers.

In the community, use of masks and good hygiene were encouraged; public gatherings were restricted; quarantines were implemented; and churches, schools, workplaces, meeting places, theaters and pool halls were closed. Masks were made by women in the community at the direction of the Red Cross. Creative alternatives to usual practices were developed, including banking by mail, and there was a great increase in use of the telephone, telegraph and Rural Free Delivery of mail. Then as now, compliance with precautions varied around the country, and some objected to masks and quarantines. In Philadelphia, on September 28, a big parade was held to promote government war bonds. Many thousands attended and became infected. Ultimately twelve thousand residents died as a result. In contrast, a parade cancellation in St. Louis at the same time is credited with a much lower death toll there.

In Europe, soldiers were badly affected by the pandemic. Prisoners of war even more so because of confinement. Mayo staff serving in France reported that the German prisoners "received the same attention and care as was given to our own men."

Armistice Day came on November 11, 1918. Like elsewhere in the country, Rochester erupted with a huge spontaneous celebration on Broadway. Attendees broke all the isolation rules, crowding and hugging and kissing. The event ended in disaster when a traffic marshal was killed by a speeding celebrant. Unsurprisingly, it was followed by a large increase in influenza cases in December and January.

It is estimated that 500 million people (one-third of the world's population) were symptomatically infected, with up to 50 million deaths worldwide. Death tolls varied around the world; 0.5 percent of the total population in the United States, 1 percent in Latin America, 1.5 percent in Africa, up to 3.5 percent in Asia, 10 percent in Tahiti, 20 percent in Western Samoa and 72 out of 80 inhabitants (90 percent) of Brevig Mission, Alaska. In the United States, the death toll from the flu was 675,000 (total population 103.2 million; 195,000 in October alone). This was nearly six times the death toll from World War I (116,516). More U.S. soldiers died of influenza in World War I than of battle injuries. In Minnesota, 11,000 influenza deaths were three times the death toll from the war (3,607). In Rochester, 360 patients were hospitalized, including 18 nurses, and 41

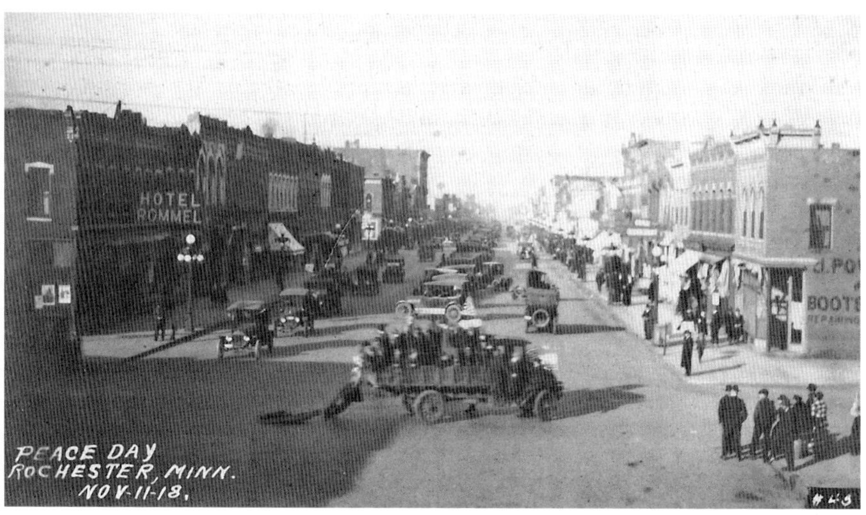

Postcard of Armistice Day celebration on Broadway.

died, including 6 Sisters of St. Francis.[98] My great-uncle William Joseph "Bill" Scanlon (Maurice's younger brother) died of influenza at the age of twenty-five in St. Aignan in the Loire Valley of France on October 30, 1918, twelve days before the armistice was declared.

The Fair, 1919

The first fair for Minnesotans occurred in 1853 when an exhibit of products from the Minnesota Territory was shown at the New York World's Fair held in the Crystal Palace. It included photographs of Fort Snelling and St. Anthony Falls, an Ojibwe birch bark canoe and other native artifacts, wild rice, fine furs provided by Henry Sibley's American Fur Company in Mendota, superlative farm products and a young wild bison bull. The historical account by William G. Le Duc, the commissioner for the Minnesota exhibit, details his trip to New York City with the bison bull. It is hilarious.[99] The Minnesota exhibit received a favorable editorial review by Horace Greeley that was thought to have stimulated the flow of immigrants to the newly settling territory.

The first Olmsted County Fair was held at the courthouse in 1860. In 1861, the Executive Committee of the Olmsted County Agricultural Society identified a forty-acre parcel of land on the north side of the Zumbro in what is now Soldiers Field. The lot was enclosed by a fence, and a half-mile racetrack was created, along with wooden buildings for exhibitions. County fairs were held there in 1861–65 despite the war. The Minnesota State Fair was held in Rochester in 1866, '67 and '69 and again in 1880, '81 and '82. Special trains were scheduled from surrounding towns. The fair attracted so many visitors that the trains were unable to provide coaches for all the passengers. Some were forced to travel in freight cars.

At the time, southern Minnesota had far greater agricultural output than parts farther north and had reasonable cause to expect to host the primarily agricultural state fair. The Southern Minnesota Fair Association was formed in 1882 with that intent. But politics dictated otherwise; the state fair never returned to Rochester. In 1885, the state fair acquired its permanent site in St. Paul when Ramsey County donated its 210-acre poor farm, the first being held beginning September 7, 1985. The fair then ceased to move from year to year. In his *History of Olmsted County*, Leonard complained bitterly: "The developments of the State fair as a grand show for the benefit of St. Paul and Minneapolis, at the expense of the whole State and supported by liberal appropriations by the Legislature, composed of a decided majority of country members, has done much to deprive such rural counties as Olmsted of their natural advantages as agricultural show grounds."[100]

The county fair remained popular, but when the Fair Association and county commissioners scheduled a vote to approve a small tax in support of a mortgage on the fairgrounds, it was defeated by 81 percent against in December 1899. Leonard commented, "The voters were willing to go to a fair but not willing to pay a cent apiece in taxes to perpetuate it."[101] The last straw for the fair came the following August. A horse racing meet was held over four days. Although the Rochester area at that time was renowned for breeding fast horses, the racing failed to draw enough spectators to be profitable. The Fair Association voted to sell the fairgrounds late in 1900 and disband. The local market for racehorses vanished. From 1901 to 1909, the county fair became a "school fair" held downtown.

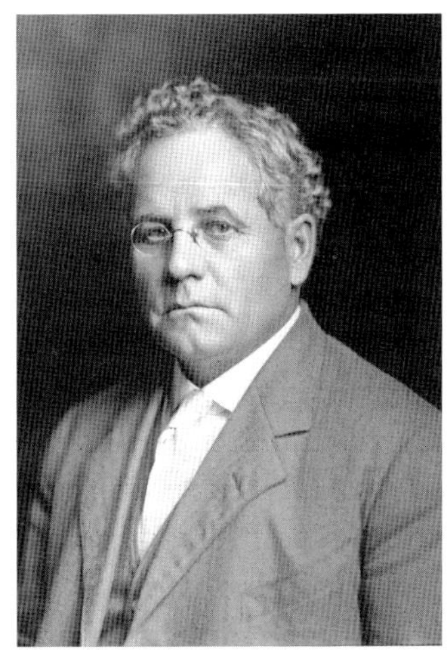

Dr. Christopher Graham. *By permission of Mayo Foundation for Medical Education and Research.*

In 1910, Dr. Christopher Graham singlehandedly revived the Olmsted County Fair by providing a different parcel of land, the current Graham Park Fairgrounds, as a new site for the county fair. He also provided several buildings and funds to support the Fair Association. In 1919, he transferred ownership of the new fairgrounds to Olmsted County, contingent only on continued use of the land for the annual county fair. It has continued most years since, with a few exceptions for wars and pandemics.[102]

Soldiers Memorial Field Park

Soldiers Field was proposed in 1924 as a public park with recreational facilities for youth that would encourage amateur athletics and would be dedicated to honor soldiers of all wars. American Legion Post 92 bought 160 acres from Dr. Christopher Graham that included the previous fairgrounds. Dr. Graham agreed to a sale price of $33,000 and accepted a down payment of $3,000. The Legion started development of a golf course in 1925. The golf course opened on May 8, 1927, as a six-hole course with sand greens. In 1927, the Legion transferred the property to the City of Rochester to be developed as a comprehensive recreational area. The golf course was expanded to nine holes and then eighteen, with grass greens. The first golf pro was hired in 1929. The property was expanded with additional acquisitions in the 1930s and '40s.

In 1929, Dr. E. Starr Judd donated the field house (designed by Harold Crawford) to the city. It was later used as part of the bathhouse for the swimming pool. The pool was built in 1936 as a Works Projects Administration (WPA) project, partly sponsored by the American Legion Post using funds loaned by the Mayo Properties Association. With fifty-yard lanes, it was the largest in the state at the time. The pool was operated by the Parks and Recreation Department. The pool was very popular. The Mayo loan was paid back by 1944. Another pool was constructed at Silver Lake Park in 1958.

The football field and running track had full lighting and seating for five thousand spectators. They were owned by the Parks Department but were managed by the school district. Rochester High School football teams played their home games in Soldiers Field from 1928 to 1958. In 1953, the proposal to build a new high school in Soldiers Field was vetoed by Mayor Claude "Bony" McQuillan, necessitating construction of John Marshall on the northwest edge of town.[103]

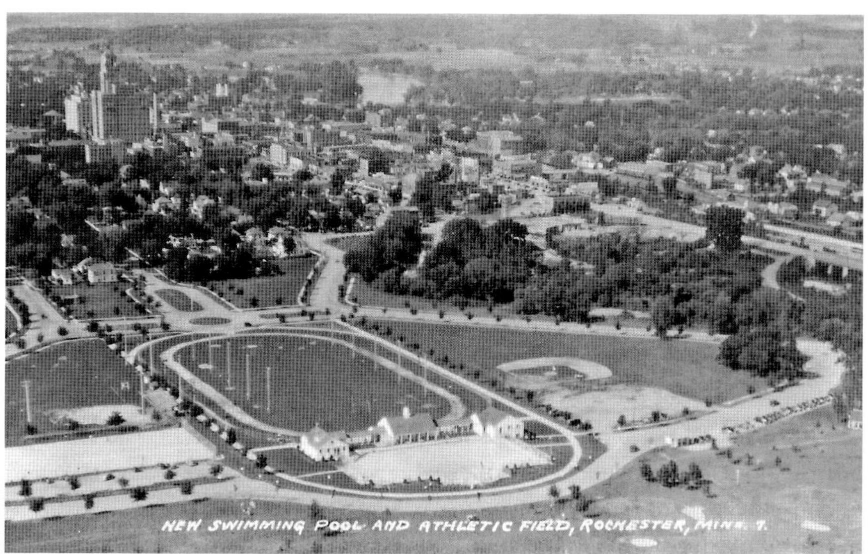

Aerial postcard of Soldiers Memorial Field.

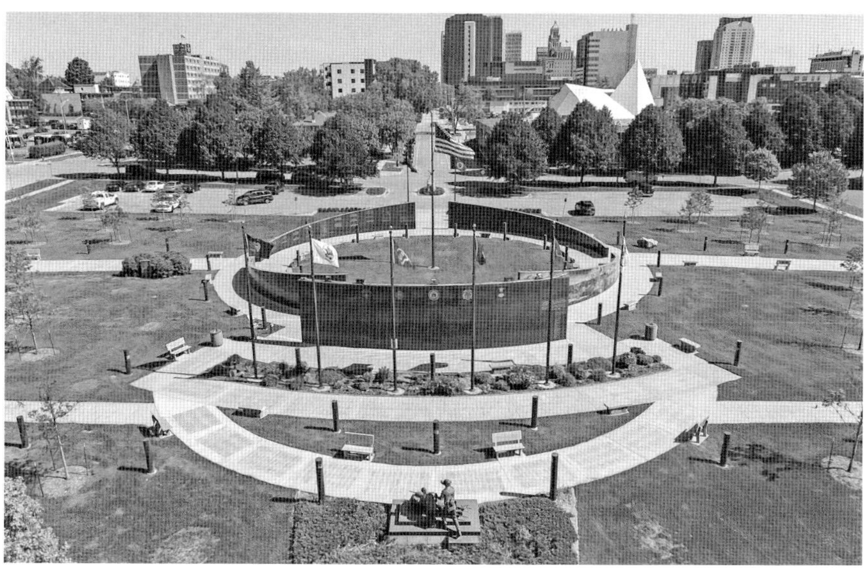

Rochester Veterans' Memorial. *Courtesy of the* Rochester Post Bulletin.

The river was extensively rechanneled in 1931. At that time, a loop of the meandering river ran as far north as the intersection of First Avenue and Sixth Street Southwest. A millpond extended southwest from there. The millrace that powered the Olds & Fishback Mill ran underground northeast from there. After recanalization, the low land in the area of First Avenue south of Sixth Street was used as a dump until 1952, when it was filled in with excavated material from the construction of the Mayo Building, bringing it up to its current level.

A modest Legion Memorial was installed at the north entrance to the park in 1951 (north of the running track and the pool). It consisted of an eagle-topped memorial and plaque, flagpole and cannon from World War I. The concept of a more extensive Veterans' Memorial began in 1965, with the Rochester Jaycees adoption of the 173rd Airborne Brigade, making Rochester the second city in the nation to adopt a Vietnam fighting unit. In 1995, the 173rd Airborne held its reunion in Rochester. The importance of the city's patronage to unit morale was apparent and inspired the idea to memorialize the 173rd. That idea was expanded to include all U.S. Armed Forces veterans from every significant conflict from the Civil War to the Gulf War. The Veterans' Memorial is privately funded though built on parkland. It is managed jointly by a committee of volunteers in cooperation with the Rochester Parks and Recreation Department.[104]

KAHLER AND METHODIST

The Cook Hotel on the southwest corner of Broadway and Zumbro Street (Second Street South) was built in 1870 by banker John R. Cook to provide the finest accommodations in the region. Sadly, the economy deteriorated, and the hotel was mostly empty in its early years. In 1886, Henry Kahler and his son, John Kahler, took over management. The economy had improved by that time, partly due to the expanding Mayo practice. They remodeled and more than doubled the number of rooms and made a success of the former white elephant. At one point, when St. Marys was fully occupied and awaiting expansion, Dr. Will convinced John Kahler to convert some of his available rooms to hospital rooms and an operating room. This established the precedent for a downtown hybrid hotel with hospital functions. That model was followed by Kahler facilities for the next sixty years, helping to accommodate the relentless growth of the Mayo practice.

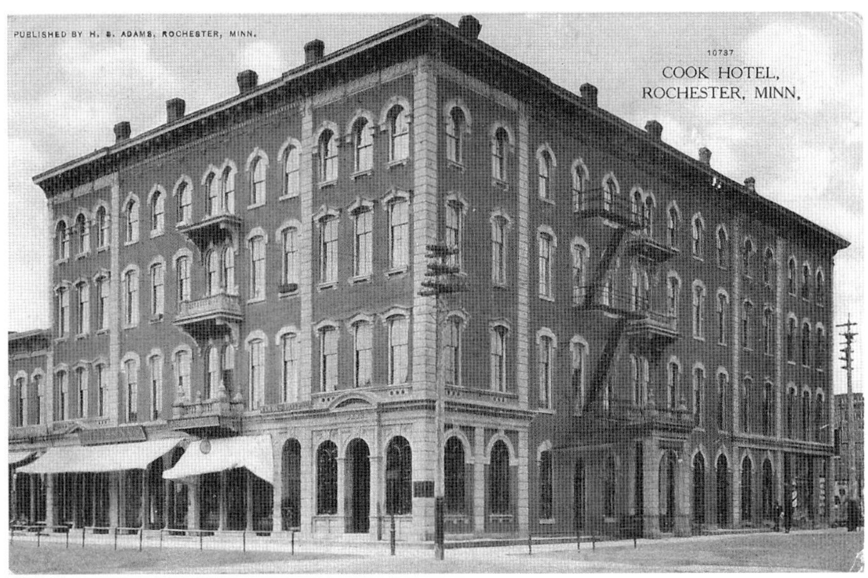

Postcard of Cook Hotel.

Several years later, in response to continued need for convalescent quarters for patients, Dr. Will convinced Mr. Kahler to build a new hotel.[105] With financial backing from the Mayos and local businessmen, they began with the residence of E.A. Knowlton, originally built for J.D. Blake, which served as lobby and front of house. They built around it a four-level T-shaped addition with hotel rooms to the south and west. The main entrance was on Franklin (Second Avenue Southwest) at the corner of Fifth Street (Center Street). It was called simply "The Kahler." It opened in 1907 and was immediately successful as the premier hotel in town. It provided sixty hospital beds in addition to hotel rooms and convalescent rooms. Two physicians provided full-time in-house medical coverage for patients and hotel guests. Kahler and co-investors went on to develop more downtown hybrid hotels, including the Zumbro Hotel in 1912 and the Colonial Hotel in 1915. The latter was repurposed before it opened and was named the Colonial Hospital, with exclusively hospital services. The Kahler Corporation was created in 1917 and proceeded with construction of three more hospitals in as many years—the Stanley (for medical services), the Worrall (ear, nose and throat and pediatrics) and the Curie (radium therapy and diet kitchen)—with a total of three hundred beds and five operating rooms.[106]

A newer, much larger Kahler opened across First Avenue Southwest in 1921 (at which point the original Kahler was renamed Hotel Damon in

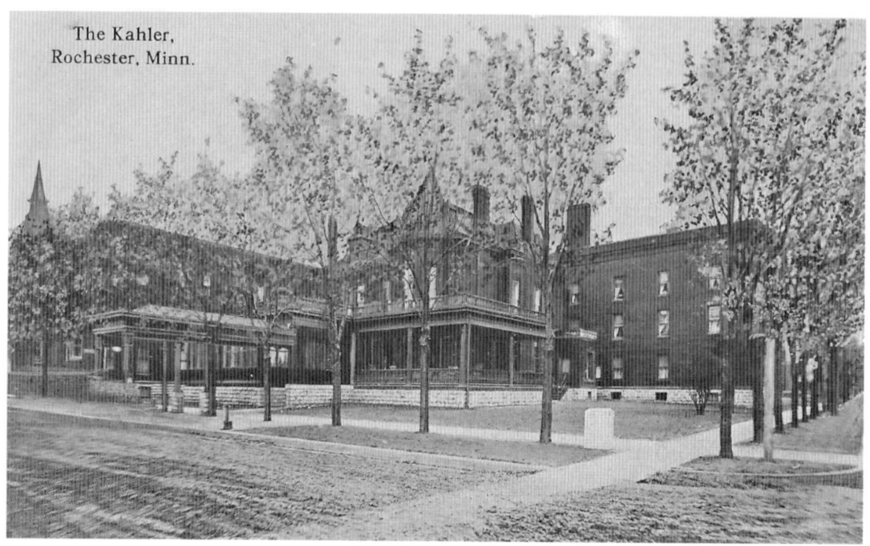

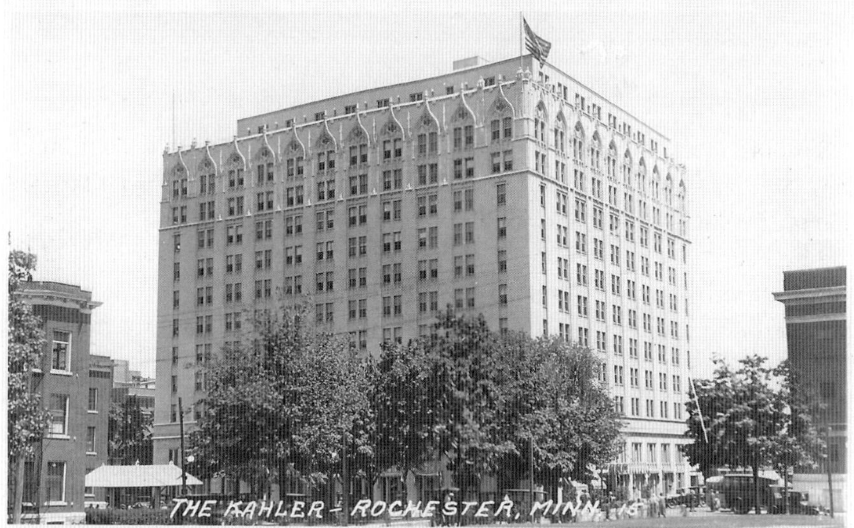

Top: Postcard of the Kahler, later Damon Hotel.

Bottom: Postcard of Kahler Hotel.

honor of Dr. Will's wife, Hattie Damon Mayo). The new Kahler's Tudor Gothic architecture was matched by elegant interior design features. Six lower floors had 220 hotel rooms. Above that were five floors with 210 hospital beds; operating rooms for oral, plastic and general surgery; and a 150-bed convalescent unit. In 1954, a major addition to the Kahler included

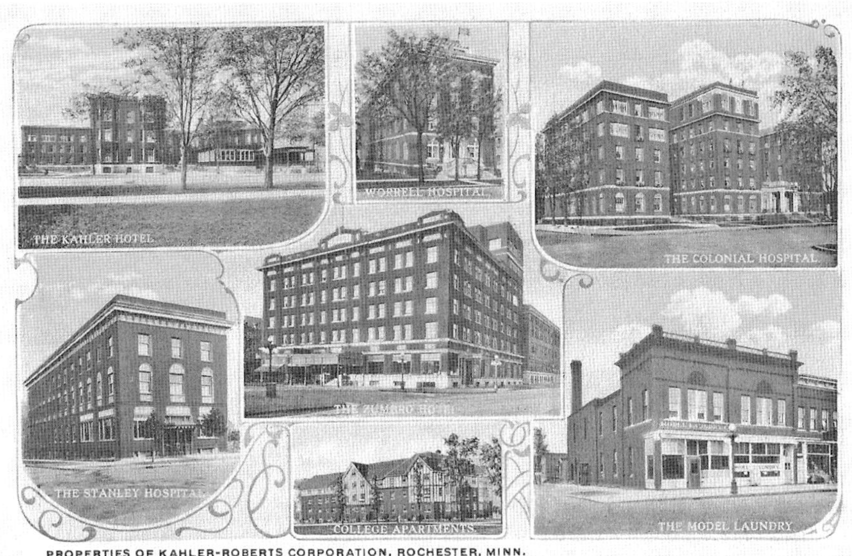

Postcard of Kahler Properties.

228 rooms on the north end. In 1968, 152 rooms, a parking garage, ground-level commercial space and a penthouse-level pool were added on the east side of the building, completing a one-block footprint.

The Kahler has been considered the finest hotel in town for most of its one hundred years. In addition to premier accommodations, the Kahler provided fine dining with a series of iconic restaurants, most notably the Elizabethan Room just off the main lobby and the Pinnacle Room on the eleventh floor. It also provided several noteworthy bars, including the Top of the Rock on the eleventh floor and the Lord Essex on the main level. Many famous guests stayed at the Kahler, including Presidents Dwight Eisenhower (when he was General Eisenhower), Lyndon Johnson, Ronald Reagan and George H.W. Bush; Vice Presidents Hubert Humphrey and Dan Quayle; King Faisal of Saudi Arabia; King Hussein of Jordan; Governor Arne Carlson; evangelists Billy Sunday and Billy Graham; television host Ed Sullivan; actors Jimmy Stewart, Randolph Scott and Fred MacMurray; boxer Muhammad Ali; baseball manager Leo Durocher; comedians Jack Benny and Danny Kaye; entertainer Marie Osmond; musician Art Garfunkel; and many others.

Grand old hotels attract ghost stories, and the Kahler is said to have its own ghost. Helen Voorhees Brach was a wealthy widow from Chicago. After

Colonial Hotel, Rochester, Minn.
American Plan. Rates $2.00 to $3.00 per day.

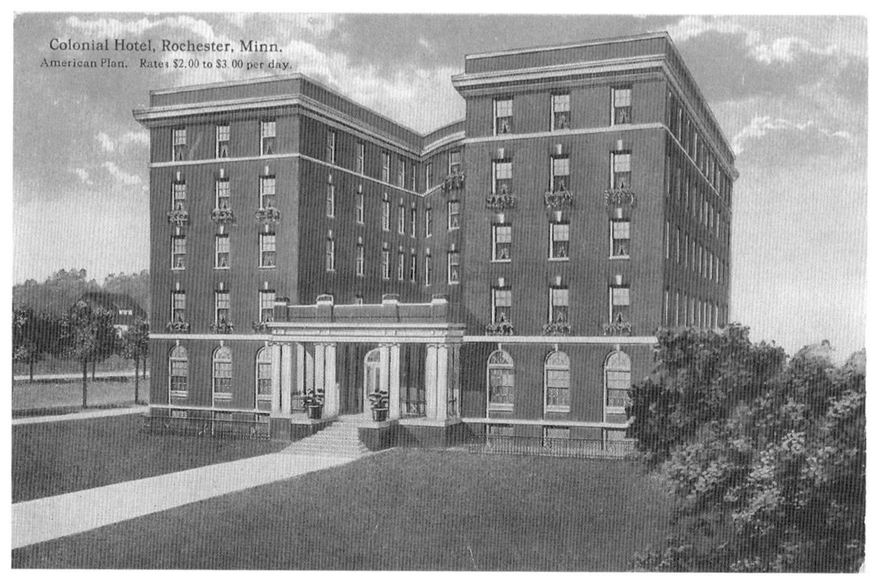

Postcard of Colonial Hotel/Hospital.

a clinic visit in 1977, she checked out of the Kahler to fly home to Chicago. She was never seen again, and her body was never recovered. She was thought to have been murdered by a Chicago crime gang in a dispute over a racehorse. Over the years since then, a number of employees and guests have reported seeing a woman on an elevator who fits her description and who disappears before their eyes.[107]

Kahler Corporation continued its dual missions, running both hospitals and hotels until 1953. At one point, there was a proposal to build a large new Kahler Hospital (see postcard image on facing page). In 1953, Kahler Corporation concluded that its for-profit hospital model was no longer economically viable. It sold all of its aging hospital facilities to the newly created not-for-profit Rochester Methodist Hospital (RMH). RMH was created through the joint efforts of the Methodist Church, notably Ralph L. Jester and Dr. Gerald and Billy Needham, and representatives of Kahler Corporation and Mayo Clinic, notably legal counsel Harry A. Blackmun, who was later a U.S. Supreme Court associate justice.

Planning for the new hospital took ten years and included the creation in 1957 of an experimental radial hospital unit, funded by the Ford Foundation and the Louis W. and Maud Hill Foundation. The innovative radial design was incorporated into nursing units on the east end of the hospital with more traditional linear units at the west end. Construction began on August

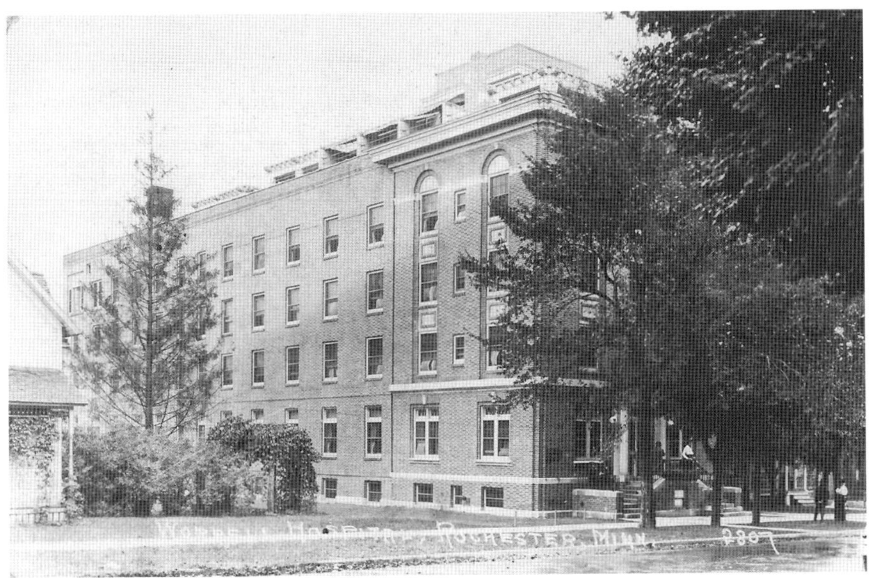

Postcard of Worrall Hospital.

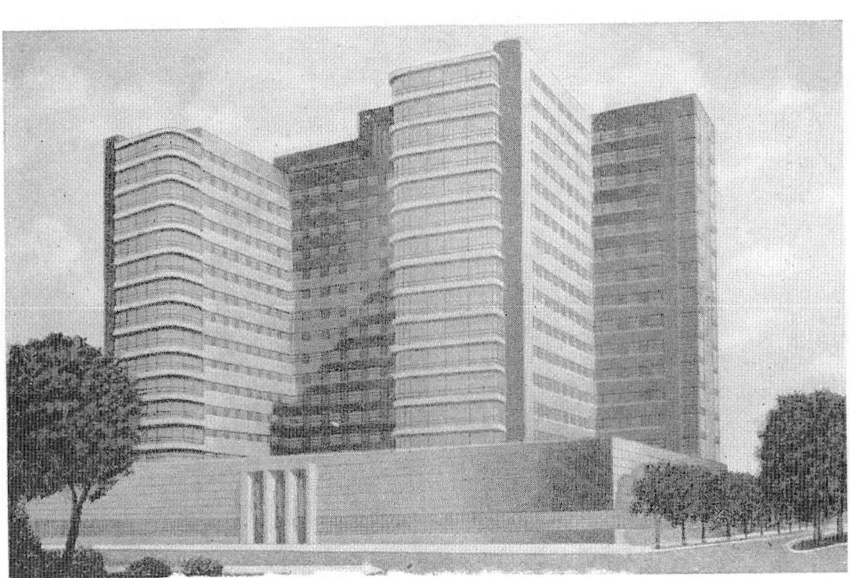

Postcard of proposed Kahler Hospital.

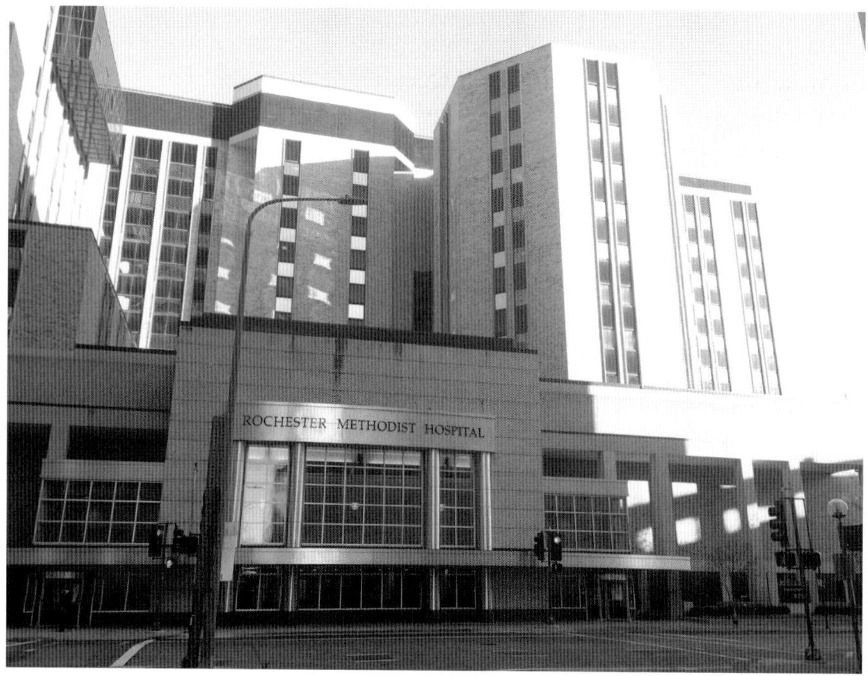

Entry of Rochester Methodist Hospital.

10, 1963. The main building is twelve stories tall and initially extended from the rear of the old Colonial along Center Street nearly to Third Avenue. Construction was complicated by the dramatic collapse of a giant tower crane on October 8, 1964.[108] With a 55-foot tower and 130-foot boom, it was the largest crane of its type in the world. When it collapsed, four iron connectors snapped, allowing the tower and boom to tip over. Fortunately, no one was killed, and only two workers received relatively minor injuries. Construction was only briefly delayed to replace a concrete slab punctured by the falling counterweight of the boom. Other cranes were available to finish the remaining stories. The new hospital was dedicated on October 21, 1966, with 30 operating rooms and 570 beds in 23 nursing stations. With additions, it grew to 990 beds.

Three of the four wings of the Colonial were razed to make way for RMH needs. One wing remains. The Damon Hotel was demolished in 1960, and the Damon Parkade and Curie Pavilion were built in its place (on the current site of the Gonda Building). Radiation Oncology moved to the new Curie Pavilion in 1963. The old Curie Hospital (on First Street between First and Second Avenues Southwest) was torn down to allow for eastward expansion of the Kahler. The Worrall Hospital and Annex were razed in the early 1970s to make way for the Hilton and Guggenheim Buildings. The Stanley was demolished and replaced with a parking garage at First Avenue and Second Street Northwest. The Zumbro was torn down in 1987 and replaced with the Kahler Plaza Hotel, since renamed the Rochester Marriott Mayo Clinic Area.

In addition to the radial unit, innovations credited to Methodist Hospital include some of the first open heart operations by Dr. John Kirklin in 1955, using the Mayo heart-lung bypass machine; the first total hip joint replacements by Dr. Mark Coventry in 1969; and development of the unit dose for medications, which set a national standard for safety and efficiency. RMH remained independent until 1986, when the Methodist Hospital Board and the Sisters of St. Francis both transferred ownership of their respective facilities to Mayo Clinic to achieve more efficient operation as a single entity. It was renamed Mayo Clinic Hospital, Methodist Campus. Included in the exchange was Charter House, a premium retirement living facility, which was relatively new and had not yet achieved financial stability. Mayo Clinic had greater resources to absorb its transient operating losses for several years, until it was more fully occupied.

In 1989, the main hospital building was named in honor of George M. Eisenberg, a Chicago businessman and philanthropist and Mayo Clinic's greatest benefactor up to that time.[109]

Nobel Laureates—Count 'em—Five!

Most Rochester residents are aware that Edward C. Kendall and Philip S. Hench (with Tadeus Reichstein of Switzerland) were awarded the 1950 Nobel Prize in Physiology or Medicine for the chemical characterization and the use of cortisone to treat rheumatoid arthritis. Kendall had isolated thyroxine, or thyroid hormone, in 1914. Drs. Howard F. Polley and Charles H. Slocumb were key members of the team as well, though they were not recognized by the Nobel Committee.[110]

Very few locals, though, are aware that five Nobel laureates called Rochester home. Only one (Hench) was a Mayo Clinic physician.[111]

Frank B. Kellogg received the Nobel Peace Prize in 1929. Kellogg Middle School is named in his honor, but few in Rochester know his first name or what he did. He was born in New York in 1856 and grew up on a farm fifteen miles from Rochester. Like Henry Wellcome, he lacked resources but

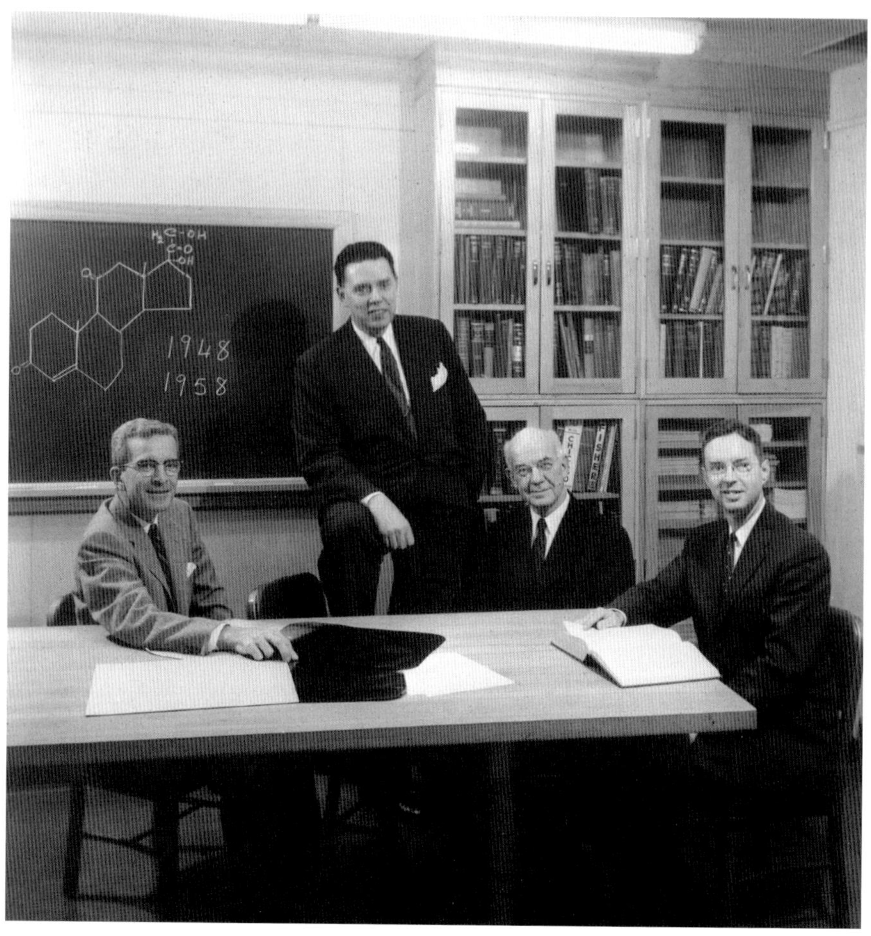

Drs. Slocumb, Hench, Kendall and Polley, structure of cortisone on blackboard. *By permission of Mayo Foundation for Medical Education and Research.*

showed intellectual promise and was encouraged and mentored by W.W. Mayo. He studied law and practiced in Rochester from 1877 to 1887. He moved to St. Paul in 1886 and became a federal prosecutor in 1905. Under Teddy Roosevelt, he was the top "trustbuster" who reined in Standard Oil Corporation and other monopolistic companies. In 1912, Kellogg was elected president of the American Bar Association, and then in 1916, he was elected to the U.S. Senate from Minnesota. President Coolidge named him ambassador to Great Britain in 1923 and then U.S. secretary of state from 1925 to 1929. At the State Department, he authored the Kellogg-Briand Pact, which was endorsed by over sixty nations, making it a crime to start a war. It was the legal basis for the prosecution of German and Japanese leaders after World War II. He was awarded the Nobel Peace Prize in 1929.[112]

Almost no one knows about Albert Szent-Györgyi de Nagyrápolt. He was born in Budapest, Hungary, in 1893. He received his PhD in 1929 from Cambridge, with an interest in cellular metabolism. He worked in Kendall's lab in 1929–30 to isolate large quantities of what he called hexuronic acid from adrenal glands. He subsequently proved that hexuronic acid is vitamin C (ascorbic acid) and discovered the catalytic role of vitamin C in Krebs cycle. He was awarded the Nobel Prize in Physiology or Medicine in 1937 "for his discoveries in connection with the biological combustion process with special reference to vitamin C and the catalysis of fumaric acid."

Likewise, very few know that Nobel Physics Laureate Luis Alvarez was once a Rochester resident. A separate story describes his achievements in section 3.

The Chateau, 1927

Movie houses had a period of opulent design before the Great Depression in 1929. The Chateau Theater is a period piece of that era. Originally called the Chateau Dodge, it opened on October 26, 1927, with the movie *Spring Fever* and a gala event sponsored by local merchants. *Dodge* was an acknowledgement of the prior business on the property, the Dodge Lumber Co. The theater was designed by the Ellerbe Firm of Minneapolis. Thomas Ellerbe, son of the founder, Franklin, was the principal architect. The Chateau was owned and operated by Finkelstein and Rubin Theaters of Minneapolis. A groundbreaking ceremony was held on April 1, 1927, with Dr. Charlie Mayo wielding a silver shovel as 1,500 people attended. Heffron and Fitzgerald were the general contractors and completed the project in only seven months, opening October 26, 1927. The facility was an "atmospheric playhouse" with a façade resembling a French château and a brilliant sunburst marquee. The lobby was evocative of a fourteenth-century medieval castle with high-beamed ceilings and wrought-iron ornamentation. The auditorium seated 1,487 in tiered seating and a small balcony. It is surrounded with silhouettes of castles with balconies, turrets, stained-glass windows, fountains and arched gateways. The ceiling had decorative lights to simulate the twinkling starry sky seen from the courtyard of the castle,

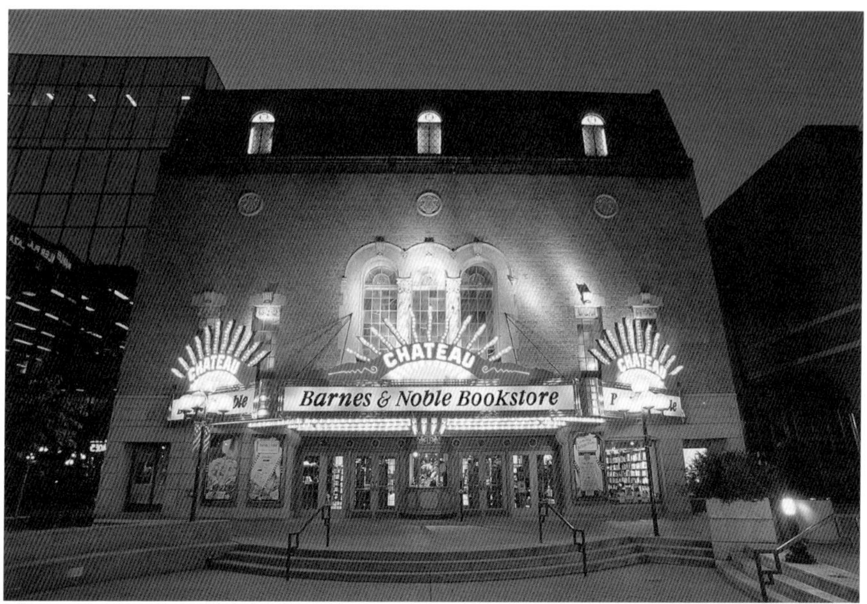

Façade of the Chateau. *Courtesy of Dean Riggott Photography.*

while the proscenium was designed to resemble the gateway to a medieval city. The theater was designed to present vaudeville acts, road shows, operas and motion pictures.[113]

The Chateau was added to the National Register of Historic Places in 1980. It showed movies until 1983. When it closed, it was threatened with demolition, prompting a Save the Chateau movement. Barnes & Noble bought the building and operated it as a bookstore from 1994 until January 2, 2015, when once again the building was threatened with demolition. The City of Rochester bought it for $6 million in 2015. Mayo Clinic contributed $500,000 toward the purchase. In 2019, the city selected Exhibits Development Group to provide exhibits along with musical performances and other events.

Subway? Where's the Train?

In 1926, as plans were beginning for the Plummer Building, a problem was recognized regarding the reliability and administrative burden of multiple utilities in support of multiple buildings of both Mayo Clinic

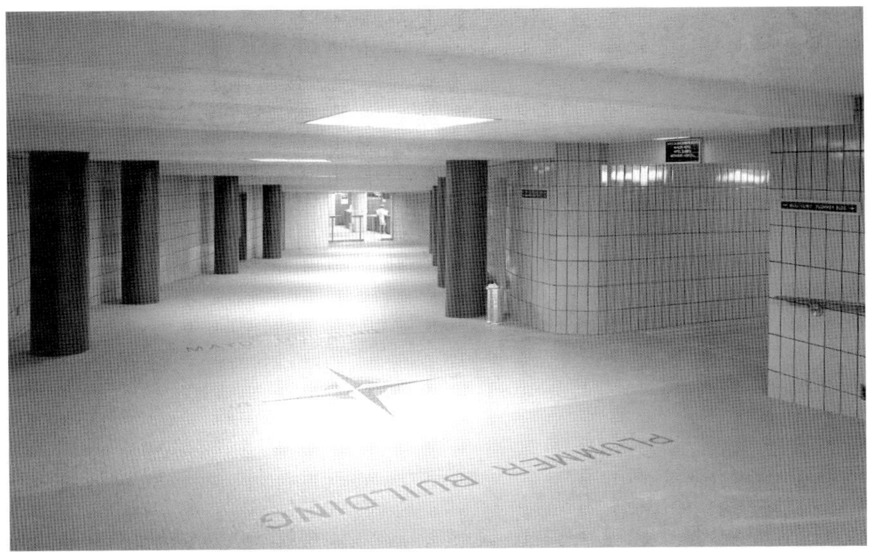

Subway intersection, 1965. Mayo Building and Medical Sciences ahead, Plummer behind, Franklin and Worrall to left and Kahler, Zumbro, Damon/Curie and Methodist to right. *By permission of Mayo Foundation for Medical Education and Research.*

and Kahler Properties. At the suggestion of Ellerbe engineers and Dr. Henry Plummer, the two entities agreed to build a single large facility, the Franklin Heating Station, to provide utilities for fifteen buildings. As they planned excavations to distribute steam lines, water lines, power lines and telephone lines to all of these facilities, the concept of utility tunnels emerged. It was then suggested to add tunnels for subterranean pedestrian traffic among the buildings. It was decided to build parallel double subterranean tunnels with utilities in one tunnel and pedestrians in the other. That design became the Mayo/Kahler pedestrian subway system, which is still in use.[114]

Dr. Chuck

Charles William "Chuck" Mayo was born on July 28, 1898. The elder son of Dr. Charlie and Edith Graham Mayo, he grew up as the second eldest of six living children (two died in infancy), plus two younger adopted siblings. Chuck attended Central School in Rochester and then Hill School in Pottstown, Pennsylvania, graduating in 1917. He received his bachelor's

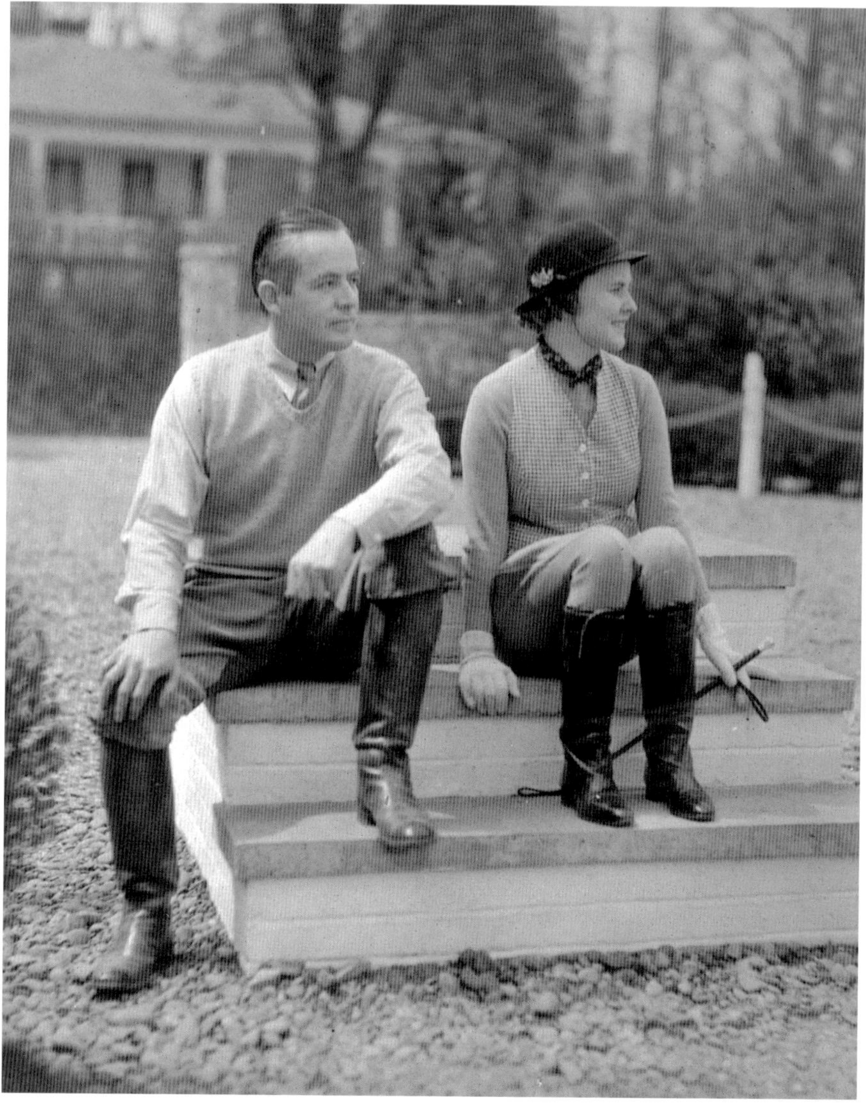

Dr. Chuck and Alice Mayo, circa 1936. *By permission of Mayo Foundation for Medical Education and Research.*

degree from Princeton in 1921, his MD in 1926 from the University of Pennsylvania and a master's degree in surgery from the University of Minnesota in 1931.

Dr. Chuck joined the staff of Mayo Clinic in 1931. Like his uncle Will, he specialized and innovated in abdominal surgery. He was particularly interested in the surgical treatment of colo-rectal cancer. He served on the Mayo Clinic Board of Governors from 1933 to 1963. During World War II, he served in the United States Army Medical Corps, attaining the rank of colonel as commander of the 233rd Station Hospital in New Guinea and then the Philippines. He was a professor of surgery at University of Minnesota and served on the University Board of Regents from 1951 to 1968, as chair from 1961 to 1967. He served as a member of the U.S. delegation to the United Nations, appointed by President Eisenhower, along with many other state, national and international leadership and advisory roles.

He married Alice Varney Plank in Philadelphia on June 25, 1927. They had six children, Mildred "Muff" Plank (1928–2009), Charles Horace II (born 1930), Edward "Ned" Martin (1931–2017), Joseph Graham II (1933–2015), Edith Maria Donovan (1937–2016) and Alexander Stewart (born 1942). They also raised David and William James Mayo II, the two sons of Dr. Chuck's brother Joe, who was killed in an auto accident in 1936. Dr. Chuck and Alice were active participants in the community and gracious hosts at Mayowood. Because of the financial strain of maintaining the enormous mansion and entertaining a constant stream of dignitaries and other guests, they were forced to sell properties from the estate to make ends meet. In 1948, they invested in a radio station, KLER, Rochester's second, an ABC affiliate. Ownership was in Alice's name in hopes of delaying the inevitable clash with the Board of Governors about conflict of interest. When that occurred, Dr. Chuck quit the board of directors of KLER, but Alice retained ownership of the station until selling it off in 1955.[115]

Dr. Chuck retired in 1963 after thirty-two years on the staff of Mayo Clinic. This was the first time the Mayo family was not represented on the staff. His autobiography, *Mayo: The Story of My Family and My Career*, is a surprisingly candid and often humorous insider's view of the Mayo family and the clinic. It was published posthumously by Doubleday shortly after he died in 1968. It was controversial because it described disagreements that he had with other members of the Mayo Clinic Board of Governors. He died in a single-vehicle rollover accident on his seventieth birthday on County Road 104 (Sixtieth Avenue Southwest) near Salem Road, two miles west of Mayowood. He is buried on the grounds of Mayowood next to his beloved Alice, who died from multiple myeloma eight months before him.[116]

Plummer Building, 1928

The Red Brick Building was designed to serve the needs of the clinic for many years. In 1914, no one expected the practice to outgrow the facility in only twelve to fourteen years, yet it happened.

Planning for the Plummer Building began in 1924 with the Ellerbe firm. Mayo's representatives were once again led by Dr. Plummer. It was built between 1926 and 1928 and was originally called the New Clinic but was renamed in honor of Dr. Plummer when the Mayo Building was built in the 1950s. It is fifteen stories tall, plus a belltower equivalent to four additional stories. At 292 feet tall, it was the tallest building in Minnesota until the Foshay Tower was completed in 1932. It was the tallest in Rochester for over seventy years, until the Gonda Building was completed in 2001. Throughout the planning process, there was debate over the size of the project. Legend has it that Dr. Plummer met with Dr. Will the evening before construction was scheduled to begin. Dr. Will had reservations about the size of the project and asked to meet with Dr. Plummer the following noon after he finished at the hospital. Dr. Plummer called the contractor and asked him to dig the biggest hole possible by noon. The following day, when Dr. Will saw the progress, he shrugged and said to go ahead as planned.

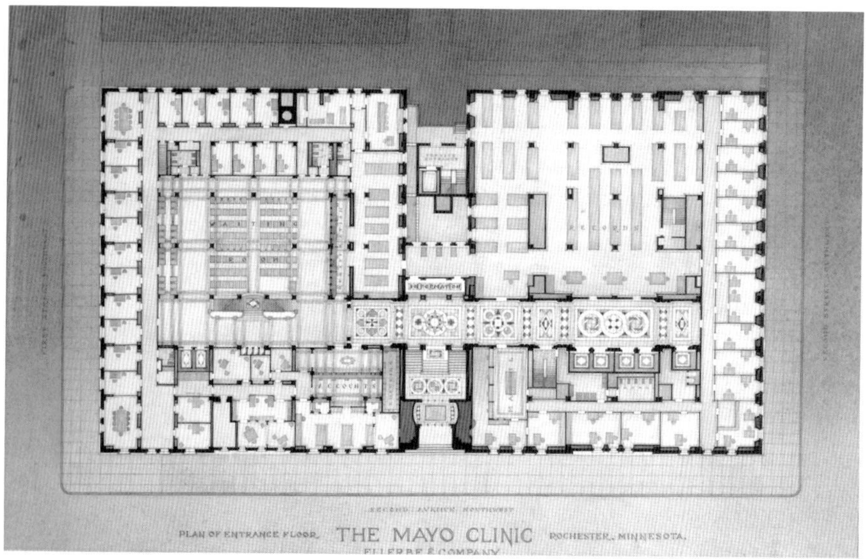

Architectural drawing of the main floor of 1914 Building and Plummer Building. This is believed to be Henry Plummer's personal copy. The stains at upper left are thought to be tobacco stains from his cigars.

The building was designed around its clinical sections and was featured in a *Life* magazine article on September 4, 1939, showing the building laid out with vertically stacked sections for registration, laboratories, radiology, general examinations, surgical consultations, dermatology, neurology, ophthalmology, pediatrics, ENT, dental diagnosis, orthopedics and so on. Over the years, spaces were reconfigured and reassigned. For example, the third floor was home to radiology until 1955, when it was assigned to clinical microbiology until 1974, then pulmonary function (PF) until 2007.

The building is a Romanesque Revival design with even greater emphasis on aesthetics than in the 1914 Building. It is built on a steel skeleton, clad in Bedford, Indiana limestone over the lower two stories and buff-colored brick above. Ray Corwin, of Ellerbe, designed the building's decorative elements. (He also designed decorative elements of the Chateau Theater and the Oakwood Cemetery gate.) The building has many carved-stone and Italian terra-cotta embellishments, including gargoyles on the belltower. The interior has hand-painted plaster frieze ceilings, terrazzo floors and Art Deco light fixtures, with quarter-sawn oak wainscoting and trim. In later years, Dr. Will reminisced, "In connection with the construction of the building, it was pleasing to note his [Plummer's] respect for the emotions of mankind and his recognition of the significance of emotional reactions. Never did the white, cold marble of the mausoleum type come into the calculations. Where marble was used, it was the warmly colored marble that would please the eye and quiet the apprehensions. In such understanding and execution of purpose Henry Plummer was perhaps at his best."

Many features of the building were state of the art, including elevators, which accounted for 10 percent of the cost of the building ($300,000 out of a total cost of $3 million in 1928); central vacuum; air conditioning; a state-of-the-art phone system; overhead paging; a light system for locating physicians and surgeons; and a pneumatic tube system for immediate transport of medical records and laboratory specimens.

The belltower was added after the fact. Dr. Will was traveling in Belgium and England and became enamored of bells. He bought a twenty-three-bell carillon from the foundry in Croyden, England. The largest bell weighs 7,840 pounds. Dr. Will informed the engineers responsible for the Plummer, which was still under construction. They managed to accommodate the late addition of the 18-ton carillon, plus the massive belltower, which were not in the original plan. Images from the time show the addition of the steel skeleton of the belltower to the building, with the brick façade already completed. The Mayos gave the carillon as a gift to the City of Rochester.

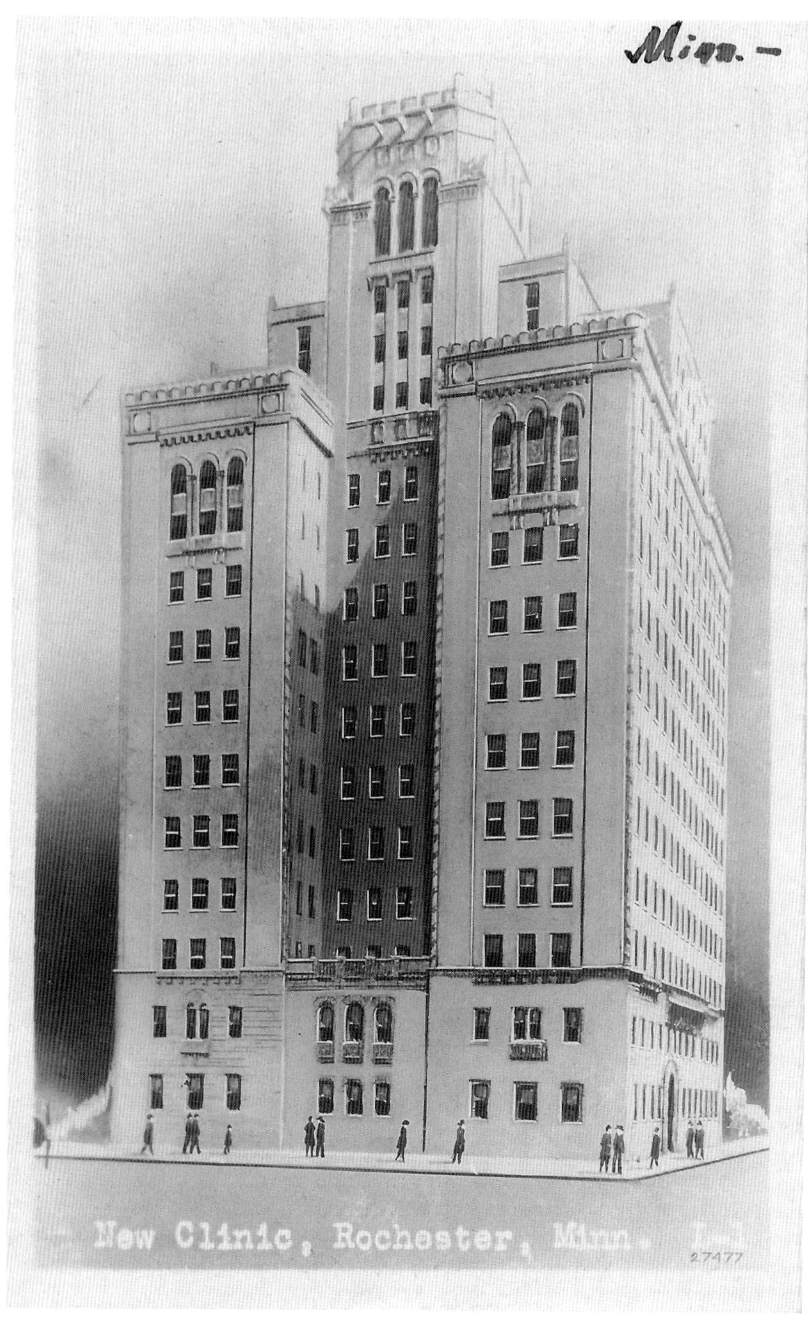

Postcard of a model of the Plummer Building before addition of Carillon tower.

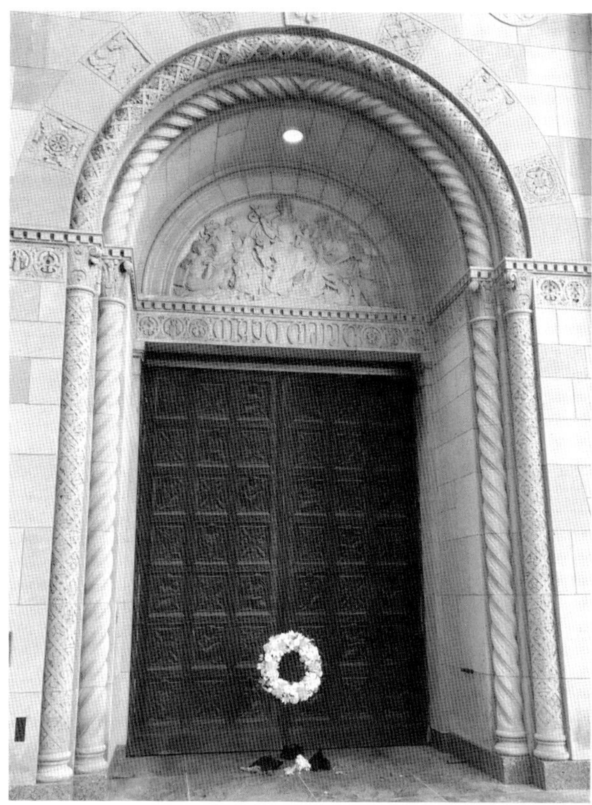

Plummer doors closed in memory of Sister Generose Gervais, October 18, 2016.

The bells were consecrated by the Archbishop of Canterbury before they were shipped from England. The largest bell is embossed, "To the American Soldier." Dr. Will said at the dedication on September 16, 1928, "Today we dedicate this carillon to the American Soldier, in grateful memory of heroic action on land and sea to which America owes her liberty, peace, and prosperity. Let the music of these bells ever remind us of our brave defenders." A gift to Mayo Clinic in 1977 added thirty-three more bells to complete a fifty-six-bell, four-and-a-half-octave carillon.

Since its inauguration there have been only four carillonneurs at Mayo Clinic: James Drummond (1928–58), Dean Robinson (1958–2004, forty-six years), Jeffrey Daehn (2004–2016) and Austin Ferguson (2017–present). Mayo Clinic is the only medical center in North America with a carillon. The Mayo Clinic carillonneur is one of only six full-time carillonneur positions in North America.[117]

The massive bronze doors were designed by St. Paul sculptor Carlo Brioschi. They are sixteen feet tall, five and a half inches thick and four thousand pounds each. The illustrated panels depict themes of Minnesota lore and motifs of education, maternity, agriculture and domestic, mechanical and fine arts, each personified as a mythological figure. The doors are kept open and have only been closed for ceremonial purposes on eleven or twelve solemn occasions: the death of E. Starr Judd in 1935 (perhaps); the deaths of Henry Plummer in 1936, William J. Mayo in 1939, Charles H. Mayo in 1939, Donald C. Balfour in 1963, President John F. Kennedy in 1963, Charles W. Mayo in 1968 and Harry J. Harwick in 1978; as a memorial to the victims of September 11, 2001; as a memorial to the victims of the Mayo Clinic helicopter crash in 2011; the death of Sister Generose Gervais in 2016; and as a tribute to the Black Lives Matter movement on July 29–30, 2020.

Joseph Fritsch was a Mayo Clinic employee for forty-five years, from 1920 to 1966. During most of that time, he served as a door attendant for the Plummer main entry. He was affectionately known as "Joe Clinic" and was renowned for both his personable manner and his remarkable memory for patients' names and faces.[118]

I joined the Mayo Clinic staff in 1984, assigned to the Pulmonary Function Lab on Plummer third floor. Sadly, the Plummer Building was in neglected condition. The brick exterior was worn, and the mortar was cracked. The terrazzo floors were cracked in many places. The plaster frieze ceilings had extensive water damage and were covered with acoustic ceiling tiles. Most of the Art Deco light fixtures had been replaced with ugly fluorescent fixtures. The beacon light that once capped the Plummer Building had been removed when the airport was moved in 1961, but the ugly aluminum gantry on which it was mounted remained on the belltower. After Craig Smoldt became the chair of the Department of Facilities, restoration of the Plummer Building started, and it was gradually returned to its former beauty. The exterior was repaired with complete tuck-pointing and repair of damaged decorative elements. The belltower was restored where it was structurally weakened. One of the bells was cracked. It was recast in England from the original mold and replaced. The cracked terrazzo floors were repaired. The plaster frieze ceilings were painstakingly repaired and repainted by hand. The original light fixtures were placed back in their original locations and upgraded appropriately with contemporary wiring and LED bulbs. Subsequent remodeling was designed to preserve and restore original features. The restoration was crowned at the suggestion of the current CEO, Dr. Gianrico Farrugia, by replacing the giant terra-cotta finial at the top of the belltower. The original was not preserved, but the plans for the original were available, and the company that produced it was still in business seventy-five years later, so it was remanufactured.[119] The Plummer Building remains the most iconic element of the Rochester skyline and a key visual identity of Mayo Clinic.[120]

The Ear of Corn Water Tower—The "Corn Cob"

A distinctive water tower in the shape of an ear of corn dominates the sky over southeast Rochester near the intersection of South Broadway and U.S. Highway 14 (Twelfth Street). Built in 1931, the tower is 149 feet tall. The tank, in the shape of an ear of corn, is 49 feet tall and holds fifty thousand gallons. It was designed by the Chicago Bridge & Iron Co., with the correct number of rows of kernels (sixteen). It has been owned sequentially by Reid-Murdoch; Monarch Foods; Libby, McNeil & Libby; and, since 1982, Seneca Foods. Until the Rochester Airport was moved in 1961, the tower marked the glide path approach to the airport from the northwest. It has been a distinctive feature of Rochester for ninety years.

Seneca closed the plant in 2018, with plans to demolish the water tower. Preservationists rallied and persuaded the Olmsted County commissioners to claim the condemned tower. In 2019, the county agreed to purchase the eleven-acre site (adjacent to Graham Park, the "fairgrounds") with factory and water tower for $5.6 million. The building has been razed, and plans are to be developed for the property while preserving the water tower as a unique landmark.[121]

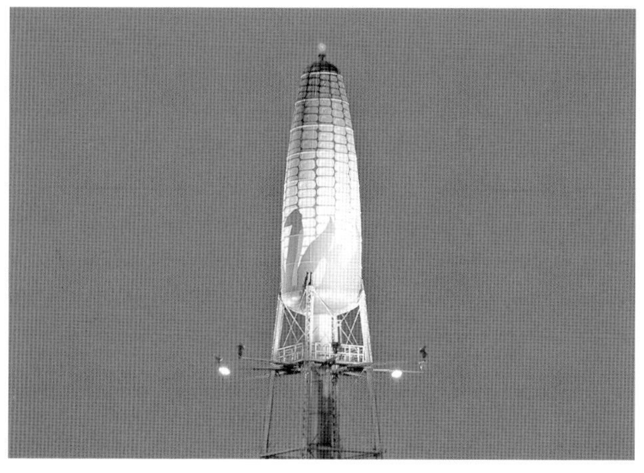

Ear of Corn Water Tower, the "Corn Cob." *Courtesy of Dean Riggott Photography.*

FDR

Franklin D. Roosevelt visited Rochester twice as president. On August 8, 1934, a blistering hot day, he presented a National American Legion citation to Drs. Will and Charlie Mayo before an estimated crowd of 125,000 (more than five times the population of Rochester at the time) in a ceremony at Soldiers Memorial Field Park.[122] The large bronze plaque reads, "American Legion Citation to William James Mayo, Charles Horace Mayo....For distinguished services to our sick and disabled comrades and to suffering humanity. The gift of William T. McCoy Post No. 92. Presented by Franklin Delano Roosevelt, President of the United States, at Rochester Minnesota, August 8, 1934." The plaque is permanently displayed on the north wall of the foyer of the Plummer Building. In 1938, the president and the first lady spent three days here when their eldest son, James, underwent surgery at St. Marys Hospital.

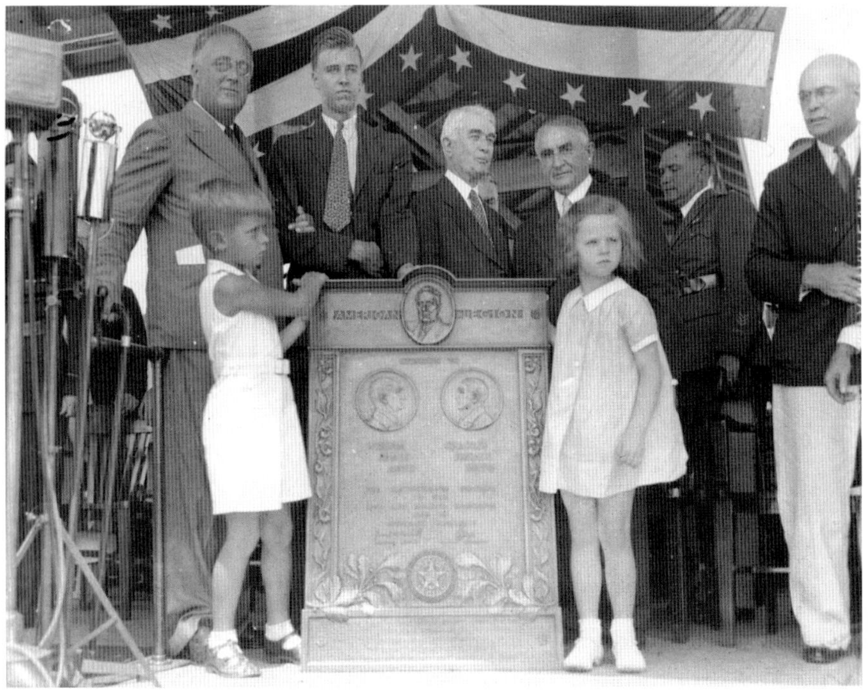

FDR with Mayos at Soldiers Field. Grandchildren "Muff" Mayo and Waltman Walters are with the plaque in front. *By permission of Mayo Foundation for Medical Education and Research, photo by Earl Irish.*

The Depression

The Great Depression began with a stock market crash. The Dow Jones Industrial Average reached a high of 381.17 on September 3, 1929, after which it lost value. On Black Thursday, October 24, 1929, it declined 9 percent in a single day. It continued to lose value until July 8, 1932, when it reached 41.22, an 89.2 percent loss from its peak. Between 1929 and 1933, unemployment increased by 25 percent and wages fell 42 percent.

Rochester was not immune to the Depression. Several federally funded construction projects were sponsored by various agencies to bolster the local economy and provide employment. They included the Works Progress Administration (WPA), the Public Works Administration (PWA), the Civilian Conservation Corps (CCC) and the Civil Works Administration (CWA). According to the *Post Bulletin*, "During the 1930s and 1940s, both the WPA and CCC brought much-needed work to locals. They improved parks and streets, built public works facilities and planted many of the trees still growing in the area. The local fairgrounds served as a headquarters for the WPA, and was the focus of some of the CCC's work."[123] Buildings include the Graham Park Heritage Sites, including Floral Hall, which is now the home of the Winter Farmer's Market and hosts many events every year, as well as buildings housing Olmsted County Fair Board, the beer garden and the blacksmith shop. "All four buildings were constructed by the WPA with stone from a quarry in southeast Rochester."[124]

The fourth Rochester post office occupied the block bounded by Center and First Street Southwest and Third and Fourth Avenues (current site of the new Damon Parkade). It was designed by Harold Crawford in 1932 and built as a CCC project. In addition to its characteristic architecture, it contained the WPA-funded mural titled *The Founding of Rochester*, painted by David Granahan in 1937. It depicts George Head driving an oxen team pulling a log to establish the right-of-way of Broadway (see image on page 17). When the post office was demolished in 1978, the mural was salvaged on very short notice by Brad Linder, director of the History Center of Olmsted County at the time, and installed at the History Center, where it still hangs.

Soldiers Field Pool was built as a WPA project in 1936. It was the largest swimming pool in the state.[125] With this facility, Rochester was a powerhouse of swimming in the state throughout my childhood in the '50s and '60s under Evar Silvernagle (twelve team state swimming championships, two hundred wins and ten losses). He taught me to swim.

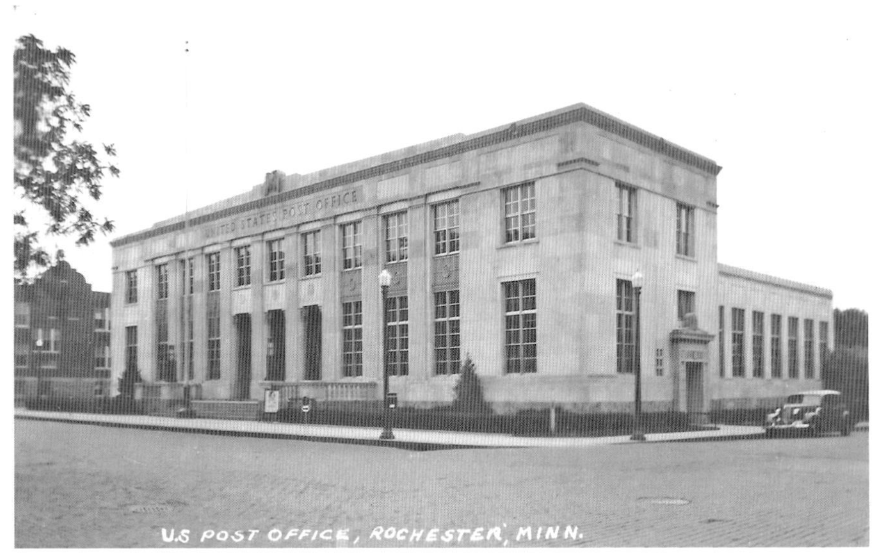

Postcard of the Depression-era post office.

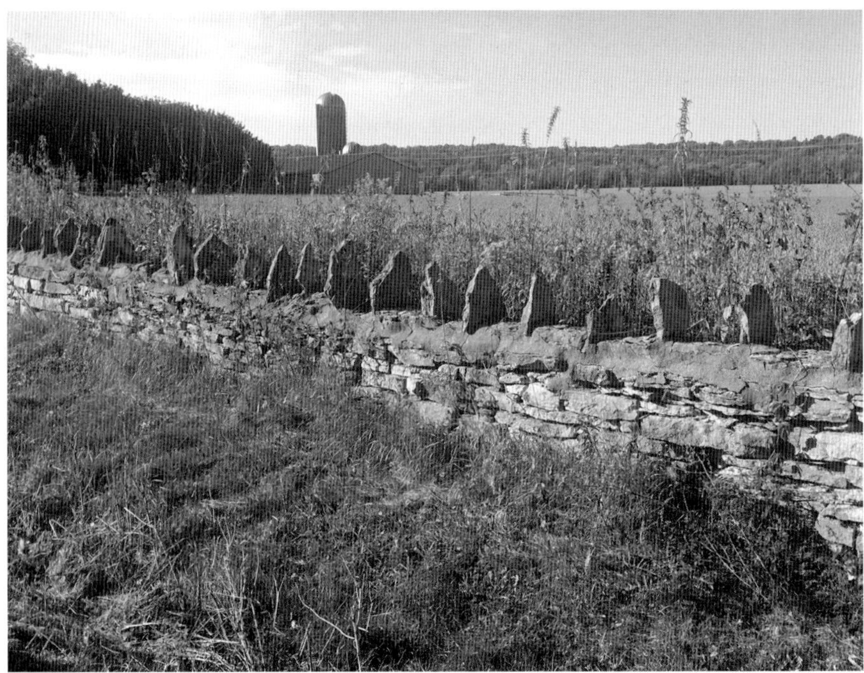

Mayowood stone wall.

The second Public Library Building at the southeast corner of Second Street and Third Avenue Southwest was a PWA project, designed by Harold Crawford in 1936 and built between 1937 and 1938 Broadway (see image on page 82). It replaced the original public library at the southwest corner of First Avenue and Second Street Southwest. Crawford designed the new building in a Jacobean style. It was built with Kasota limestone. The PWA grant funded 45 percent of the building costs, and the remainder was funded by the Library Board. It had a capacity for seventy-five thousand books, with a children's section in the lower level and adult books on the upper two levels. In the 1970s, the public library moved to larger, though less elegant, quarters at the vacated JCPenny building at the northeast corner of South Broadway and First Street Southeast. Mayo Clinic bought the vacated building, and since 1972, it has functioned as the Mitchell Student Center of Mayo Clinic Alix School of Medicine. It provides a library/resource center, administrative offices, computer facilities, classrooms, meeting space and recreational space for medical students. It has been listed in the National Register of Historic Places since 1980.[126]

Other employment during the Great Depression was provided by Dr. Charlie Mayo, who hired out-of-work men to build miles of decorative and functional limestone walls along the roads leading to his estate at Mayowood. They stretched from Sixteenth Street Southwest along both sides of Mayowood Road and from the Highway 52 exit onto Salem Road Southwest all the way to Mayowood, approaching from either Bamber Valley Road or the northwest entrance to Mayowood at the end of Mayowood Road, a total over ten miles in length. These walls were still present, intact and functional during my childhood in the 1950s but sadly have been damaged or removed outright in all but a few places. Their original form, with the "dragon's tooth" caps, is best preserved at the west end of the straightaway approaching Mayowood Stone Barn.

Silver Lake

Silver Lake is named after Silver Creek, which enters the Zumbro River just south of Seventh Street Northeast. It was created as a Works Progress Administration (WPA) project during the Great Depression. The bed of the South Fork of the Zumbro was excavated north of downtown during the winters of 1936–38, and a dam was built in 1936 to create a lake upstream

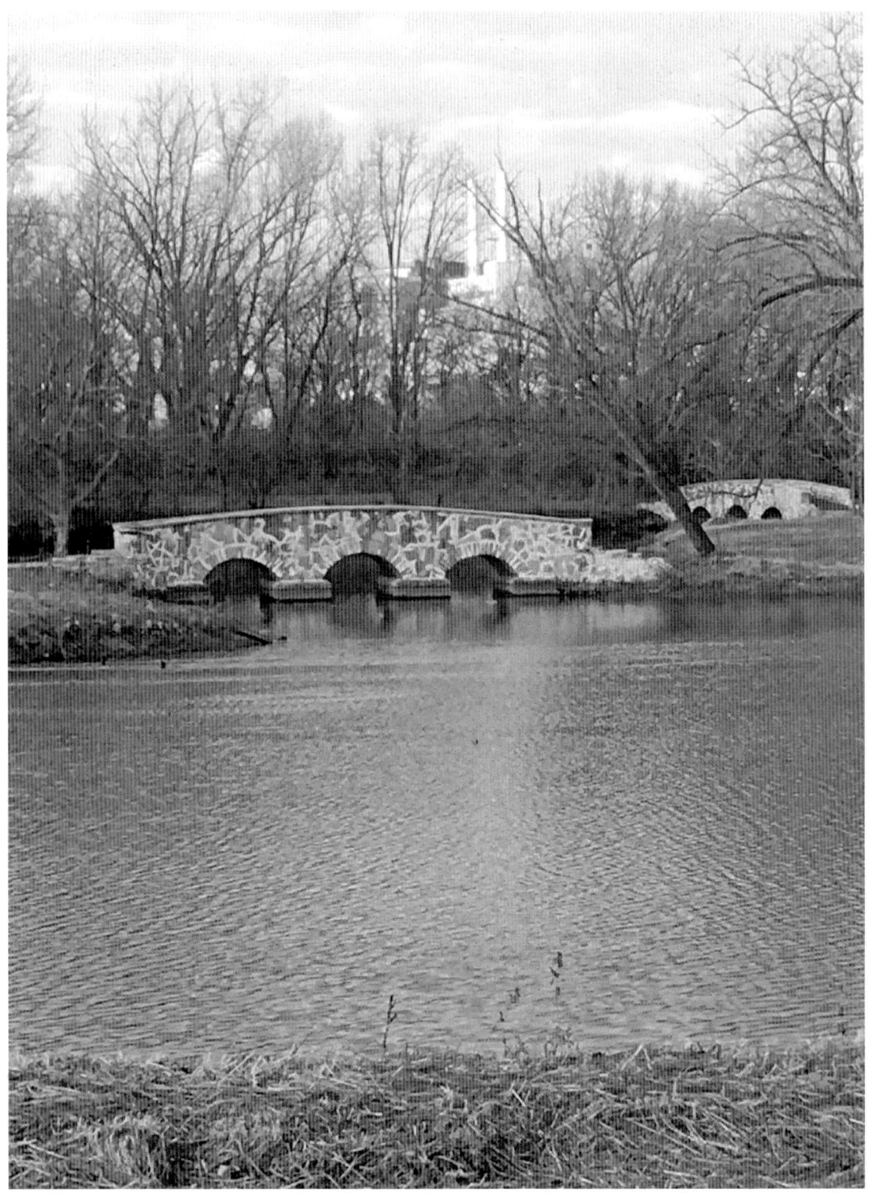

Bridges at Silver Lake east reservoir in late fall, with the power plant in the background.

of the crossing under Broadway. It included the creation of an east lagoon. Three photogenic arched limestone footbridges, built in 1936, provide access to an island in the middle of the east lagoon. The limestone was quarried at Quarry Hill.[127]

The Silver Lake Power Plant was built on the site of the historic millpond of Cole's Mill, which was on the site of the former Silver Lake Fire Station. Construction of the power plant began in 1947, and it began operation in April 1949. The plant ceased the use of coal for power generation in 2013 and stopped generation of electricity in 2015. It is currently used only to produce steam for Mayo Clinic. It is scheduled to cease steam production in the near future. The three-hundred-foot smokestack had not been used since the plant ceased burning coal. It was demolished in April and May of 2020. As of this writing, plans for the site have not been made, but it will leave a large tract of land in a gorgeous near-downtown location surrounded by water and parkland. It will be interesting to see how its next use is decided.

Giant Canada Geese

The giant subspecies of the Canada goose (*Branta canadensis maxima*) is larger and heavier (with a wingspan up to eighty-four inches and average weight of twelve and a half to twenty-two pounds) than its close relatives. It was thought to be extinct for over thirty years but was rediscovered in Rochester, Minnesota, in 1962 by biologist Harold C. Hanson from the Illinois Natural History Survey. He was visiting on invitation from the Minnesota Department of Conservation and the United States Fish and Wildlife Services to study the local flock of Canada geese.

In 1924, Dr. Charlie Mayo bought 15 Canada geese from a North Dakota breeder for Mayowood. They multiplied and attracted migratory geese to become resident, growing to a flock of 600 at Mayowood by 1936. In that year, the city transferred a group of 6 geese from Mayowood into Silver Lake, which was newly created. After Dr. Charlie died in 1939, the geese at Mayowood were not fed, and some dispersed to Silver Lake on their own. When the Silver Lake Power Plant was activated in 1948 and began to drain its waste hot water into Silver Lake, the open water in winter encouraged further growth in both the wintertime flock and the resident flock. The number of geese at Silver Lake in January increased from 250 in 1952 to 6,000 in 1964.

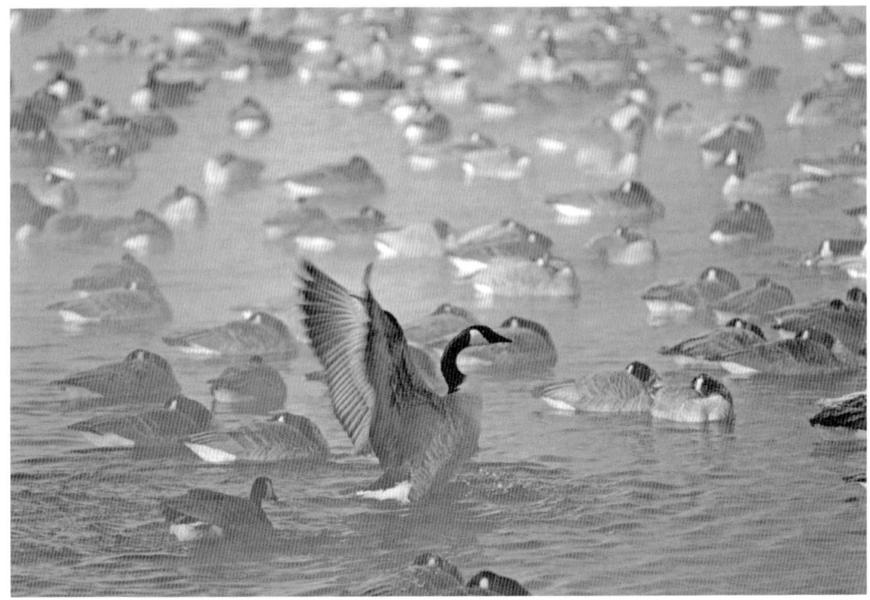

Giant Canada geese at Silver Lake. *Courtesy of Dean Riggott Photography.*

The goose population in Rochester was encouraged to grow with restrictions on hunting after 1962. The Department of Natural Resources paid local farmers to leave corn crops standing in fields for the geese. Federal migratory waterfowl protections were applied, and a generally supportive attitude among citizens of Rochester favored growth. The local goose population reached a peak of forty thousand in 2005 and spilled over to repopulate urban areas throughout North America. Other populations were encouraged by transplanting flocks of geese from the Midwest to the Eastern Seaboard, where they also flourished. The migratory population of geese summers in northern Manitoba and Ontario. Most make the five- to six-hundred-mile trip from Rochester nonstop in about ten hours.

The giant Canada goose became an icon of the city, as depicted on the city flag, in the names of a local baseball team and a popular restaurant, as well as numerous other elements of advertising and popular culture.

As the goose population grew, the perception of a nuisance also grew. This relates to abundant feces, potential for disease transmission (for example avian H5N1 influenza), traffic disruption, noise, et cetera. Mitigation strategies include discouragement of feeding geese, termination of hot water dumping in Silver Lake (reducing open water in winter), addition of lakeside buffer vegetation to restrict mobility and nesting of geese, encouraging goose hunting and liberalizing hunting regulations. These have reduced the resident goose population to between 8,500 and 10,000, although the migratory flock still numbers up to 35,000 individuals that pass through each fall until spring. Some complain that the decline in numbers has reduced the opportunity to experience the local geese. Those people have not walked through Silver Lake Park in the spring.[128]

One Million

In January 1938, Florence Lumsden of Salmo, British Columbia, was registered as patient number one million at Mayo Clinic. Registration numbers are issued serially and are permanent and unique within the entire Mayo Clinic system. Current new-patient registration numbers are greater than twelve million.

Lou Gehrig, 1939

Lou Gehrig played first base for the Yankees from 1923 to 1939. He was a great hitter and a durable player, nicknamed the "Iron Horse," with the most consecutive games played (2,130, a record that stood for fifty-six years, until it was surpassed by Cal Ripken Jr. in 1995). His career batting average was .340. He hit 493 home runs and had 1,995 runs batted in. He had the record for most career grand slams (23, since broken by Alex Rodriguez). He was an All-Star seven consecutive times, a Triple Crown winner once, an American League Most Valuable Player twice and a member of six World Series champion teams. He was elected to the Baseball Hall of Fame in 1939 and was the first major-league baseball player to have his uniform number (no. 4) retired.

Gehrig noticed fatigue and loss of muscle power in 1938, and his performance declined dramatically early in 1939. On May 2, 1939, he told his manager, "I'm benching myself, Joe....It's for the good of the team." His wife called Mayo Clinic for an appointment, which was arranged by Dr. Chuck Mayo himself. Six weeks later, Gehrig flew to Rochester for evaluation at Mayo Clinic in the Department of Neurology. He underwent six days of examinations and was diagnosed with amyotrophic lateral sclerosis, a degenerative disorder of nerves that innervate skeletal muscles. The disease has since been commonly called Lou Gehrig's Disease. He returned to New York and on July 4 gave his famous "Luckiest Man on the Face of the Earth" speech at Yankee Stadium. He died two years later, on June 2, 1941, at the age of thirty-seven.[129]

MAYO CLINIC IN WORLD WAR II

The 71st Army General Hospital was organized in Rochester in 1940 in anticipation of the war. Staff were recruited from the clinic and Rochester. In January 1943, the hospital was activated in Charleston, South Carolina, and in June, was assigned to the 233rd and 237th Station Hospitals, commanded by Charles W. "Dr. Chuck" Mayo and Dr. James Priestly. In January 1944, they shipped to New Guinea and in 1945 moved to the Philippines, where they served to the end of the war.

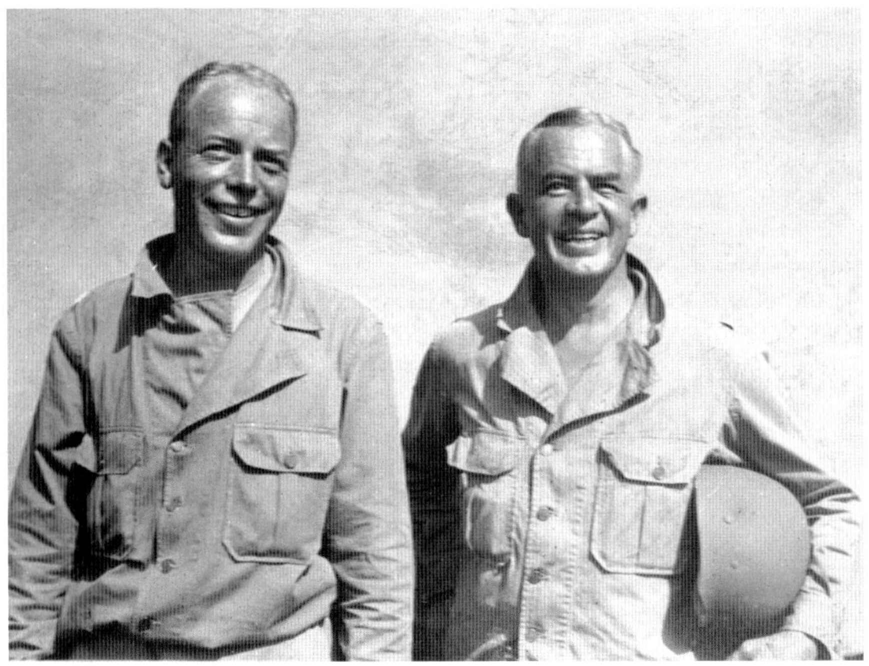

Colonels James "Jim" Priestly and Charles W. "Chuck" Mayo. *By permission of Mayo Foundation for Medical Education and Research.*

The Aero Medical Unit

During World War II, well before the United States declared war, Mayo Clinic supported the Allied war effort in many ways. Based on a secret contract between Mayo Clinic and the U.S. government, members of the Department of Physiology and others developed key technologies that were critical to military aviation during and after the war and eventually to space flight.

The first was a key solution for what was then called "oxygen want" at altitude. Barometric pressure gradually decreases as altitude increases. Human performance can decline because of oxygen lack beginning as low as seven to ten thousand feet of altitude. Exposure to altitudes above twenty-five to thirty thousand feet is quickly lethal. This can be overcome by increasing either barometric pressure or the fraction of oxygen to achieve a partial pressure of oxygen close to what is experienced at sea level. Decompression at high altitude can cause serious injury when low pressure causes dissolved nitrogen to come out of solution, forming bubbles in the bloodstream. Investigators at Mayo Clinic developed an oxygen mask named after its developers, Drs. Walter Boothby, Randolph Lovelace and Arthur Bulbulian. The BLB mask was introduced in 1938. It was initially developed for civilian aviation but was quickly adapted to Allied military needs and used during the war by U.S. pilots. In 1940, President Roosevelt presented Drs. Boothby and Lovelace with the Collier Trophy, the highest U.S. aviation award, for their work in creating the BLB mask.

Additional challenges arose from the improved performance of military aircraft. Aerial maneuvers with rapid change in direction result in the equivalent of increased gravitational force, often called "pulling Gs." Sustaining seven or more times the force of gravity can cause loss of consciousness for even the most skilled pilots. The Aero Medical Unit studied this with a human centrifuge and sophisticated monitors created for this purpose. They also performed real-world testing with test subjects sitting in the rear of a fighter plane, flying out of the Rochester Airport. The fighter plane was provided by the air force and was called the G-Whiz. The two key developments they produced were the G-suit and the M-1 maneuver. The G-suit is a tightly fitting garment with air-filled bladders to apply pressure to the limbs to preserve blood flow to the brain during rapid acceleration. The G-suit used by today's fighter pilots is very similar to the one developed at Mayo Clinic in the 1940s. The M-1 maneuver is a grunting maneuver that pilots still use today to raise their blood pressure

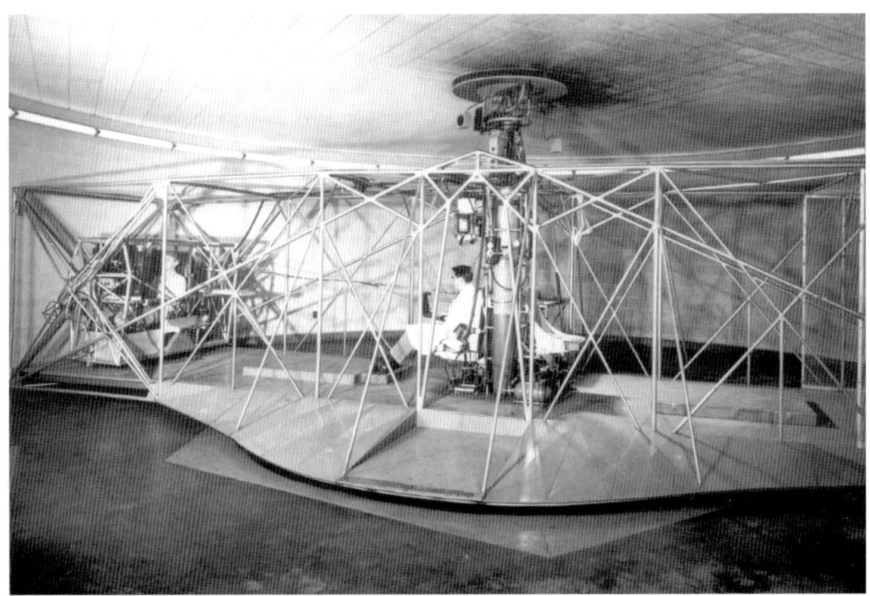

The human centrifuge in the Mayo Aero Medical Unit at the Medical Sciences Building, with Dr. Earl Wood observing. *By permission of Mayo Foundation for Medical Education and Research.*

to maintain blood flow to the brain when pulling Gs. The *M* stands for Mayo. It still goes by that name, though most people don't know the origin of the name.

A fourth major development of the Aero Medical Unit was the oxygen bail-out bottle, a small supply of oxygen sufficient to preserve life when pilots or crew were forced to bail out of their aircraft at high altitude. Dr. Lovelace, who was a lieutenant colonel in the air force, was the first to test the device in a real high-altitude maneuver. He bailed out from a record altitude of 40,200 feet. The trial was successful, but because the air was so rarified at that altitude, his speed was greater than expected. When his parachute deployed, he lost consciousness. He lost a glove in the process and suffered permanent frost injury to his hand. He was awarded the Distinguished Flying Cross for bravery.

Dr. Edward Baldes, director of the Aero Medical Unit, received a President's Certificate of Merit in recognition of his contribution to the war effort. The Aero Medical Unit was disbanded after the war, but the oximeters and other measurement devices developed for the studies had many applications in research and clinical medicine. Members of the team continued their research and made major contributions in cardiac, respiratory and renal physiology and clinical contributions in cardiovascular, respiratory and renal medicine, anesthesiology, catheterization and critical care. The human centrifuge was used for research during the early stages of the U.S. space program until the early 1970s. It was dismantled in 1978 to make room for an early high-performance computed tomography scanner called the Dynamic Spatial Reconstructor or DSR. The history of the Aero Medical Unit is documented in a short video available on the Mayo Clinic website or on YouTube: "Reaching New Heights: Secret Stories of the Mayo Clinic Aero Medical Unit."[130] Unfortunately, because the research was top secret, it was never published in the scientific literature.

Newton Holland and Rochester Art Center

Rochester Art Center was founded in 1946 in an unused room on the second floor of the old Public Library at First Avenue and Second Street Southwest. Its first exhibition, January 12–31, 1947, featured thirty-six paintings by fourteen Minnesota artists. Later, in 1948, it purchased and moved to the vacated German Methodist Church at Third Avenue and West Center Street. In that small space, it provided many events, including classes, exhibitions, lectures, demonstrations, meetings and even the first rehearsals and founding meetings of the Rochester Civic Theatre. By 1956, it had outgrown that small facility. Later that year, the Art Center leased a city-owned lot in Mayo Park on East Center Street, next to the Zumbro River. The board and members raised the funds to build an eight-thousand-square-foot, two-story building. Groundbreaking was in 1957, and it opened on March 23, 1958. It was expanded in 1965. Like the current building, it was donated to the city and in return was leased back for one dollar per year for fifty years. The city provided support for maintenance of the building while the membership and a variety of grants supported programming.

In the 1950s, it was a revolutionary concept to have an institution supporting the presentation of art and arts education in a small community. The Art Center had very strong leadership. The board chair was restaurateur Newton Holland, who expressed the mission "to join with the schools, the churches, the library and other community groups to make Rochester a cultural center worthy of its scientific achievement." He, like the Mayos, recognized the importance of the cultural amenities in the life

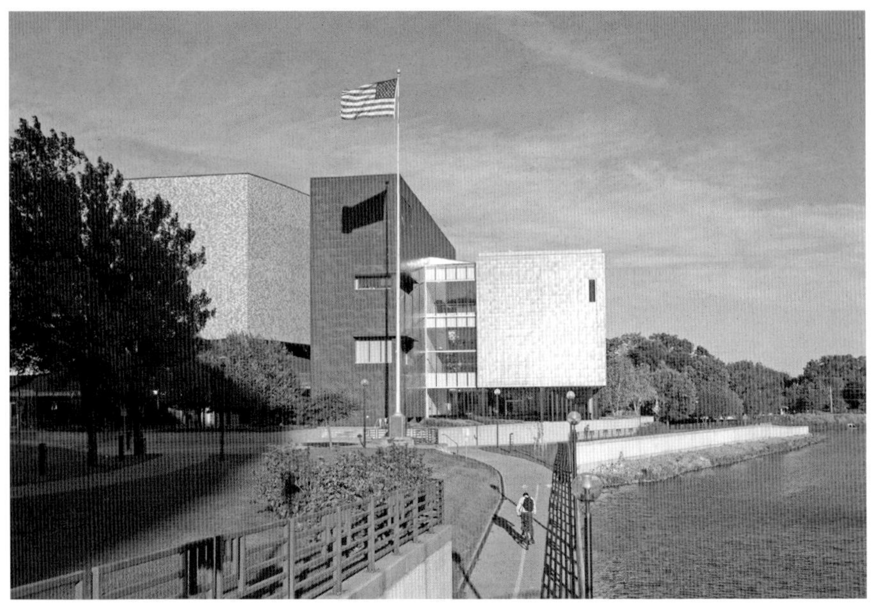

Rochester Art Center. *Courtesy of Dean Riggott Photography.*

of the community. The original board included Alice Mayo, Christopher Graham, Hiram Essex and thirteen other community leaders.

The Art Center also started out with strong professional leadership with Mr. William Saltzman, a distinguished Minnesota artist and arts educator. He served as executive director from 1948 to 1964, when he moved to St. Paul to continue his artistic career and serve on the faculty of Macalester College.

In the 1970s, B.J. Shigaki was hired as executive director (and de facto curator). Artist Judith Onofrio founded the Total Arts Day Camp educational programs while serving on the board as well. The two provided strong professional leadership for over thirty years.

In the late 1990s, an expansion of the Mayo Civic Center severely limited access to the Art Center. In compensation, the city offered alternative land at the south end of Mayo Park, as well as partial financial support toward a new building. The board launched a capital campaign in 1999. With contributions from the City of Rochester, publisher John M. Nassef, Mayo Clinic and community donors, they reached the goal of $8.2 million in 2003.

Designed by Hammel, Green and Abrahamson architectural firm with Kara Hill as lead project designer, the thirty-six-thousand-square-foot building was constructed by Market & Johnson of Eau Claire, Wisconsin, and occupied in 2004. The unique, contemporary copper- and zinc-clad buildings highlight their surroundings, including the adjacent Mayo Civic Center. The first-floor interior features a three-story atrium and grand lobby, with extensive glass windows taking in a panorama over the downtown, the Zumbro River and Mayo Park. The exhibit spaces on the second and third floors have shown the work of local, regional, national and internationally renowned artists, as well as historical and scientific exhibits. The main gallery is named in honor of renowned artist Judith Onofrio and her husband, Dr. Burton Onofrio. Educational programs that began with the Total Arts Day Camp over fifty years ago continue to provide arts education for elementary age children up to adults.

Mayo Memorial

The Mayo Memorial was initiated after Dr. Charlie's death, while Dr. Will was still alive (though he was not informed). The citizen committee first met on January 26, 1940. The large memorial plaza was to include a larger-than-life cast bronze statue of the two brothers by renowned sculptor James Earle Fraser. He described the challenge of creating the statue and the memorial: "Not only a fitting monument to the Mayos and Rochester, but it must also be of world import, because of their international fame....I believe we have found a conception which is original and beautiful. In short, a shrine where one may sit quietly and contemplate the worth to Humanity of these great brothers."

Fundraising was successful. The memorial was dedicated on September 22, 1952. The statue is 8 feet tall and depicts the brothers standing in their surgical gowns. It stands against a 13-foot-high granite backdrop on an elevated dais above tiered granite steps. It is surrounded by a 104-foot semicircular granite amphitheater. Inscriptions around the amphitheater state: "They revered the truth and sought to know it....Their rare vision still challenges tomorrow....Here they lived and worked for humanity.... Surgeons, Scientists, Lovers of their fellow men." Extending to the west was a 600-foot mall, bordered on the north by the Civic Center, on the south by the river and on the west by Civic Center Drive. At the west end of the mall was the larger-than-life bronze statue of their father by Crunelle.

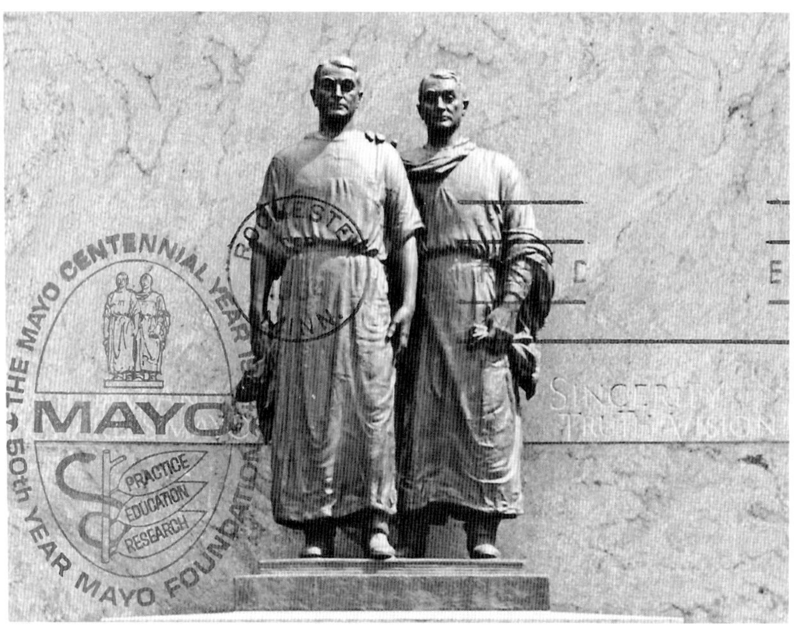

Statue of Mayo brothers by James Earle Fraser, postcard image.

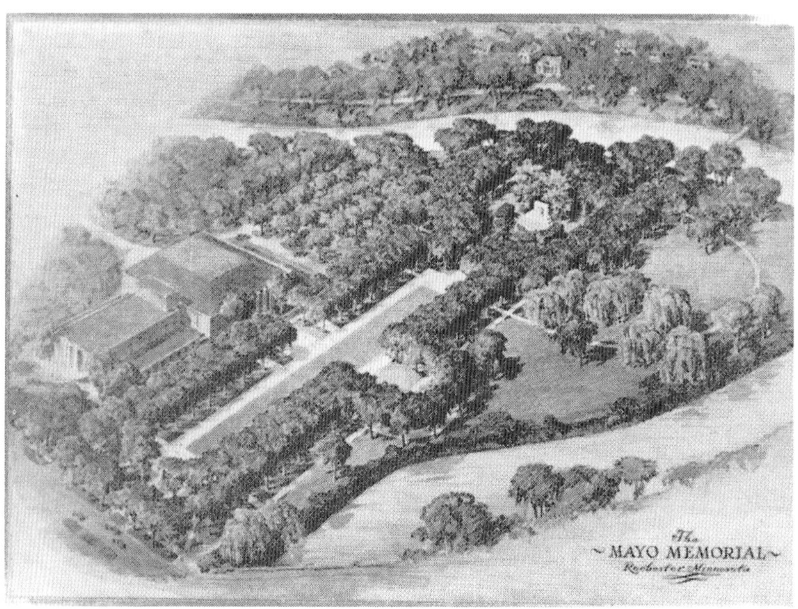

Mayo Memorial image from promotional brochure.

Over the years, additions to the Mayo Civic Center for the Arena, the Rochester Art Center and the Convention Center have filled most of the space once occupied by the mall. Several years ago, the statue of the Mayos was moved to the west entrance approach to the Civic Center. In 2015, construction of the Convention Center necessitated a move. After two years in storage, the statue was placed back in its original position on the dais of the amphitheater, where it remains, a beautiful but far less prominent display.

3
In My Lifetime

Polio, 1952

I was born in 1952, a year of pandemic polio, and retired late in 2019 at the start of the COVID-19 pandemic. Poliomyelitis, or polio, is a viral disease that, in its severe form, attacks motor neurons, the nerves that control muscles. When motor neurons are damaged or killed, the muscles they innervate become weak and atrophic. Patients with severe polio can die of respiratory failure. For unknown reasons, polio became a nearly annual pandemic in the summers of the mid-twentieth century, and 1952 was the worst year of all. Over 58,000 Americans, mostly children, developed paralytic or severe polio that year, with over 3,200 deaths and more than 21,000 who suffered some degree of long-term disability.

Polio was worse in northern latitudes and among upper socio-economic white people, so Rochester was not spared. Drinking from water fountains was discouraged. Swimming pools and beaches were closed. Public gatherings were restricted. Quarantines were implemented for the infected.

I grew up with families who suffered the consequences of the polio epidemic. Several friends and neighbors had atrophic limbs or severe scoliosis (curvature of the spine), and the mother of one friend was chronically dependent on a ventilator. She lived in St. Marys Hospital for over thirty years with chronic respiratory failure and taught generations of Mayo physicians to treat respiratory patients as real people. My medical subspecialty, pulmonary and critical care medicine, evolved in response to the need for respiratory support for victims of polio in the 1950s.

The injectable inactivated polio virus vaccine, developed by Jonas Salk, was released in 1955. The oral attenuated virus vaccine, developed by Albert Sabin, was released in 1961. I received both. I do not remember the first, but I do remember that the second, announced with great fanfare, seemed anticlimactic when I merely had to drink a sip of very sweet liquid from a tiny paper cup. The vaccines were successful, and polio became a distant memory thereafter, except for families who lived with the aftermath.

We were lucky. For over sixty years, we have not had to deal with a great pandemic, until now. Our closest encounter was the influenza pandemic of 2009, which strained the capacity of ICUs all over the world. The SARS epidemic of 2002–4 was more terrifying but fortunately was contained through heroic efforts at a handful of medical centers.

Justice Harry Blackmun

Harry Andrew Blackmun was born in Nashville, Illinois, on November 12, 1908, and grew up in St. Paul. He attended Harvard as an undergraduate math major. He graduated from Harvard Law School in 1932. He returned to Minnesota and served a seventeen-month clerkship with Judge John B. Sanborn Jr. on the Eighth Circuit Federal Court of Appeals. (Located in St. Paul, it serves Minnesota, Iowa, North Dakota, South Dakota, Nebraska, Missouri and Arkansas.) Then he worked for the firm now known as Dorsey & Whitney, with specialty interest in taxation, trusts and estates and civil litigation. He also served as adjunct faculty at the University of Minnesota and St. Paul College of Law (now known as Mitchell Hamline School of Law). In 1941, he married Dorothy Clark. They had three daughters. From 1950 to 1959, he served as Mayo Clinic's in-house legal counsel, a period he referred to as his "happiest time," in contrast to his later work as a justice, during which he said he "performed his duty." In addition to medical litigation and property law, his work at Mayo Clinic included dealing with complex organizational tax rules and vigorously defending the Mayo name from unauthorized use. (See "*Mayo v. Mayo*.") He played a key role in establishing Rochester Methodist Hospital (RMH), negotiating on behalf of both Mayo Clinic and the Methodist Church. He wrote the articles of incorporation for RMH in 1955. His wife, Dorothy, was the founding president of the Methodist Hospital Auxiliary. He served as president of the local Rotary Club. He fondly acknowledged his association with Mayo Clinic throughout the remainder of his career.

In 1959, Blackmun was urged by his childhood friend Warren Burger and Judge Sanborn to accept the nomination for Sanborn's seat on the Eighth Circuit when he moved to senior status. Blackmun agreed and was nominated by President Eisenhower. He was rated by the American Bar Association as "exceptionally well qualified," was confirmed by the Senate and received his commission on September 21, 1959. He served until June 8, 1970, during which he authored 217 opinions. In an early example of working from home, he continued to live in Rochester and maintained his office here while serving the Eighth Circuit.

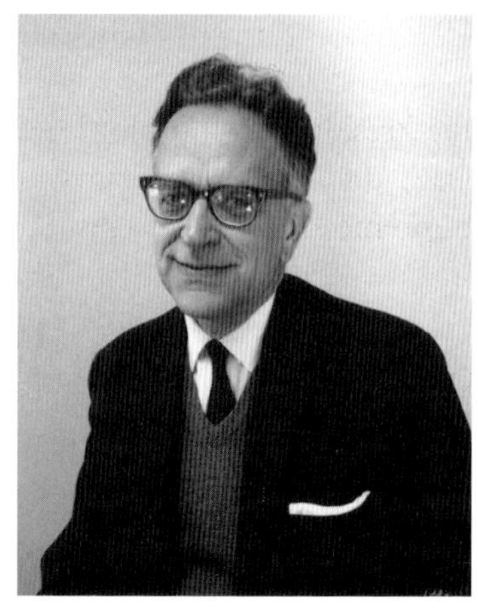

Harry C. Blackmun, legal counsel for Mayo Clinic, later associate justice of the U.S. Supreme Court. *By permission of Mayo Foundation for Medical Education and Research.*

In 1970, Blackmun was nominated to the Supreme Court by President Nixon to replace Associate Justice Abe Fortas. He was confirmed by the Senate, 94–0, and took the oath of office on June 9, 1970, at the age of sixty-one. He was best known as the author of the majority opinion on *Roe v. Wade* in 1973, in which a 7–2 majority of the court struck down a Texas law that made it a felony to perform an abortion in most cases. The decision was based on a woman's right to privacy. Blackmun wrote, "A right of personal privacy…is broad enough to encompass a woman's decision whether or not to terminate her pregnancy." He became the target of conservative backlash, including hate mail and death threats.

Justice Blackmun also made important contributions with opinions regarding affirmative action, civil liberties, immigrants' rights and commercial speech. According to Francis Helminsky, "In *Regents of the University of California v Bakke*…Blackmun contributed a minority opinion that recognized the responsibility of medical schools to consider racial and ethnic factors in admissions decisions to increase the diversity of the profession."[131] He wrote, "In order to get beyond racism, we must first take account of race. There is no other way."[132]

Blackmun and Chief Justice Warren Burger were close friends since childhood. He was Burger's best man at his wedding. They were often called the "Minnesota Twins." During Blackmun's tenure, they drifted apart philosophically, as Blackmun became more liberal in his opinions (around

1975–80), and personally, as they sometimes expressed bitter disagreements. Among Blackmun's many honors, in 1988, he was the inaugural recipient of the President's Award for Distinguished Contributions to Law and Medicine from the American Society of Law and Medicine. He retired from the Supreme Court on August 3, 1994, during the Clinton administration. He was succeeded by Stephen Breyer. He died on March 4, 1999, at age ninety, of complications of a hip fracture. After his death, at his request, a portion of his ashes were scattered on the grounds of Mayo Clinic.[133]

"Big Blue," 1956

IBM began operations in Rochester in 1956, with 174 employees working in a 50,000-square-foot leased facility. On September 30, 1958, it occupied a distinctive campus in northwest Rochester that was designed by renowned Finnish American architect Eero Saarinen, featuring a futuristic style with blue-glass-clad buildings. The corporate nickname "Big Blue" is thought to derive from the blue color once pervasive among IBM's large computers. The campus was built on 492 acres. It had 576,000 square feet (13.2 acres) of production space when it opened. At its peak around 1990, more than eight thousand employees worked in over 3.6 million square feet of space (82-plus acres) in a mile-long facility. Rochester shipped more than $500 million worth of computer hardware and electronics worldwide annually. It was the largest IBM facility in the world under one roof.

The facility started with the manufacture of punch card processing equipment. The Rochester development laboratory was created in 1961. It excelled in innovation, including the design of new computer systems, manufacturing processes, optical readers, medical applications and data storage and processing devices. The best known was the AS/400, a very popular mid-range business computer introduced on June 21, 1988. It was preceded by the successful System/3, System/32, System/34, System/36 and System/38, all Rochester products. Rochester inventors have been awarded more than 2,700 U.S. patents for product innovation. In 1990, the AS/400 Division of IBM Rochester received the Malcolm Baldrige National Quality Award, the nation's highest award for quality.

Blue Gene/L was the world's fastest supercomputer in 2004. It was developed and produced in Rochester. Since then, IBM has consistently produced some of the fastest supercomputers, including the current fastest,

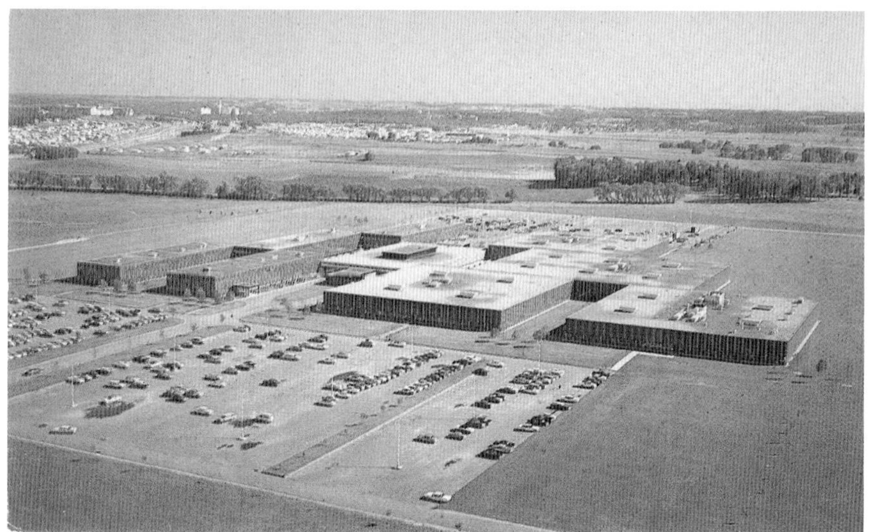

Aerial postcard of IBM Rochester plant.

called Summit. IBM Rochester had several key roles in the creation of Summit. It is located at the Department of Energy's Oak Ridge National Laboratory. It is capable of 148 petaflops. (1 petaflop is equal to 1 quadrillion, or 1 million billion, calculations per second.)

Despite Rochester being IBM's most productive plant for many years, it has been reduced in staff and space since 2000. In March 2013, the company announced further reductions in workforce as it moved several major operations to New York and Mexico. Parts of the plant have been deactivated by IBM and are now used by other technology businesses. Half of the campus was sold in 2018. Current employee counts are no longer public but are estimated to be below three thousand.

In an interesting twist, as IBM has downsized, numerous former IBM employees have started their own Rochester-based companies. This might be best personified by Al Berning, who was an engineer and operations manager at IBM from 1979 to 1994. He founded and became CEO of Pemstar, an electronics manufacturer, from 1994 to 2007 and then CEO of LiquidCool Solutions, producing cooling systems for electronics, from 2007 to 2012. Most recently, he is CEO of Ambient Clinical Analytics in cooperation with Mayo Clinic developers, supporting medical decision-making in emergency and critical care settings. Numerous other Rochester-based technology companies have key personnel who began their Rochester careers at IBM.[134]

Mayo v. Mayo

Mayo Lemon Priebe Sr. (September 1, 1900–March 30, 1978) was a local businessman. On May 2, 1957, he and two partners incorporated as Mayos Drug and Cosmetic Inc. They manufactured, packaged and sold Mayos A-Wake Tablets (caffeine 1¾ grain per tablet), Mayo-Cin (Aspirin 3 grain, Acetophenetidin 1¾ grain, Caffeine ¼ grain, MgCO3 1 grain, Al(OH)3 1 grain per tablet) and Mayos Lotion in Rochester, Minnesota, and elsewhere.

In October 1957, Mayo Clinic, represented by the Dorsey Law Firm, sued to bar use of the name "Mayo" by Priebe and his partners. Hearings began on November 25, 1957; a temporary injunction was issued on June 14, 1958; and a permanent injunction was ordered on November 10, 1959. The defendants moved for a new trial, which was denied, and then they appealed to the Supreme Court of Minnesota. The ruling by Justice Frank T. Gallagher was issued on March 2, 1962. After describing and arguing a number of points, his ruling concluded:

> *This case involves what appears to be such an obvious attempt to capitalize on a famous name known the world over for plaintiffs' developments in medical, surgical, and kindred fields for the relief of human sufferings, that it is our opinion that the order appealed from should be affirmed.*
>
> *In so affirming we are not saying that any person whether humble or famous has not the right to honestly use his own name for any business open to him.... We are, however, saying that in doing so, such a person cannot unfairly use the trade name of another or a confusing simulation thereof (even without fraudulent intent) whereby an ordinary purchaser has been or is reasonably likely to be deceived as to the true identity of the goods, services, or business, to the detriment of the plaintiff or the public, and is misled into believing that he is getting plaintiff's product when he is in fact getting that of defendant.... The test is whether the similarity is such as would deceive the ordinary customer....*
>
> *It would indeed seem naive for us to say under the record in the instant case that anyone purchasing, for example, products in a small container or bottle marked Mayo-Cin, Mayos A-Wake Tablets, or Mayos Lotion, Rochester, Minnesota, might not be deceived into believing that it was a product originating from the well-known Mayo Clinic of Rochester, Minnesota. Affirmed.*[135]

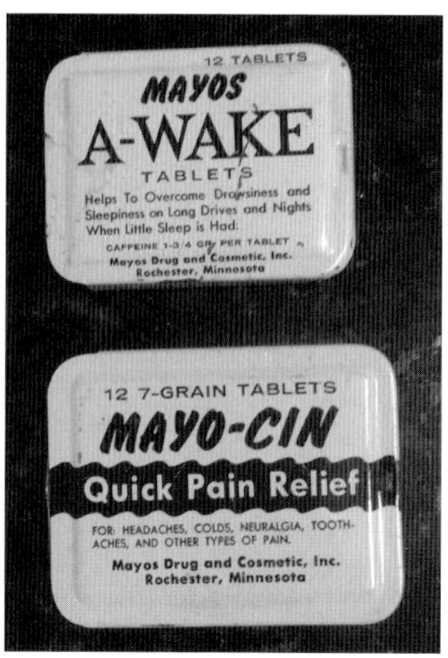

Mayos A-Wake and Mayo-Cin.

Mayo Clinic has been vigilant against misappropriation of the Mayo name, yet it is a relatively common surname. Legitimate users of the name have occasionally been confused with Mayo Clinic or the descendants of William Worrall Mayo. Examples include actress Virginia Mayo (Virginia Clara Jones, November 30, 1920–January 17, 2005), who was among the first to be honored with a star on the Hollywood Walk of Fame in 1960. Actress Edna Mayo (March 23, 1895–May 5, 1970) starred in twenty-nine silent films from 1914 to 1918. Contemporary actress and musician Miranda Rae Mayo (born August 14, 1990) has performed in numerous television series, including *Law and Order: LA*, BET's *The Game*, *Days of Our Lives*, ABC's *Pretty Little Liars* and *Blood & Oil* and since 2015 as firefighter Stella Kidd in *Chicago Fire*. Third baseman Eddie Mayo (April 15, 1910–November 27, 2006) played for the Detroit Tigers from 1936 to 1948. In 1945, they won the World Series, and he was selected to the All-Star team and was runner-up for the American League MVP Award. The Mayo Hotel has been a luxury Art Deco hotel in Tulsa, Oklahoma, since 1925. Mayo General Hospital was a large rehabilitation hospital in Galesburg, Illinois, for wounded military personnel during World War II. Although named in honor of Drs. Will and Charlie Mayo, it was a U.S. government facility unrelated to Mayo Clinic. It closed in the 1980s. USS *Mayo* (DD-422) was a World War II, U.S. Navy Benson-class destroyer named for Admiral Henry Thomas Mayo (no relation), launched on March 26, 1940, and decommissioned on March 18, 1946, after serving in both Atlantic and Pacific campaigns of the war. Mayo's Cut Plug was a brand of tobacco sold by P.H. Mayo and Brother, of Richmond, Virginia. The company was founded in 1830, and Mayo's Cut Plug was trademarked in 1878. They were among the first distributors of baseball cards.

Black and Immigrant Experiences

On July 1, 2019, the U.S. Census estimated the population of Rochester at 118,935, of which 80.3 percent are white (75.8 percent non-Latino white and 5.9 percent Hispanic or Latino); 7.8 percent are Black or African American; 7.2 percent are Asian; 3.1 percent are two or more races; 0.4 percent are American Indian and Alaska Native; and 0.1 percent are Native Hawaiian or other Pacific Islander. During most of the history of Rochester, the Black population was much smaller. In 1860 and 1870, the census showed the population of Olmsted County increasing from 9,524 to 19,766. The then-named "Colored" population increased from 0 to 27, with no "Indians" either year.[136]

The only mentions of Black people in Leonard's 1910 *History of Olmsted County* are the death of Taylor Combs at the state hospital in 1898[137] (see page 49) and the 1871 murder of James Willis,[138] a nineteen-year-old barber's apprentice. Willis, who was Black, had an argument over pay with a barber named Henry Stevens, who was white. A fight ensued in which Willis beat Stevens. Shortly after, Stevens borrowed a revolver from an acquaintance, sought out Willis and provoked another argument. Stevens shot Willis three times, killing him. He was tried and convicted of second-degree manslaughter and served four years and three months in prison.

From their beginnings, St. Marys Hospital, Methodist Hospital and Mayo Clinic offered care without regard to race, and Black patients received medical care, but no Rochester hotel and very few rooming houses were willing to provide them accommodations. Verne Manning visited Rochester with his wife for medical care in 1944 and had difficulty finding accommodations. In response, the Mannings bought the former Northwestern Hotel at 301 North Broadway. They renamed it the Avalon Hotel. Built in 1919, it had housed and fed visiting Jewish clients under the ownership of Sam and Lena Sternberg. The Avalon served clients without regard to race—the only hotel in town that did so. The Mannings were the first Black business owners and one of only six Black families in Rochester at the time. Exclusion of Blacks by all other hotels continued until it was legally prohibited in the mid-1950s, despite a 1947 Governor's Interracial Commission of Minnesota that publicly described the policies of Rochester hotels as an embarrassment to the whole state. During those years, Avalon hotel guests included Count Basie, Duke Ellington, Nat King Cole, world boxing champ Henry Armstrong and the Ink Spots.[139]

Mayor Claude H. "Bony" McQuillan (1947–51 and 1953–57) was a former professional football player and light heavyweight boxer. He was a physically imposing individual and was very popular. He was not known to

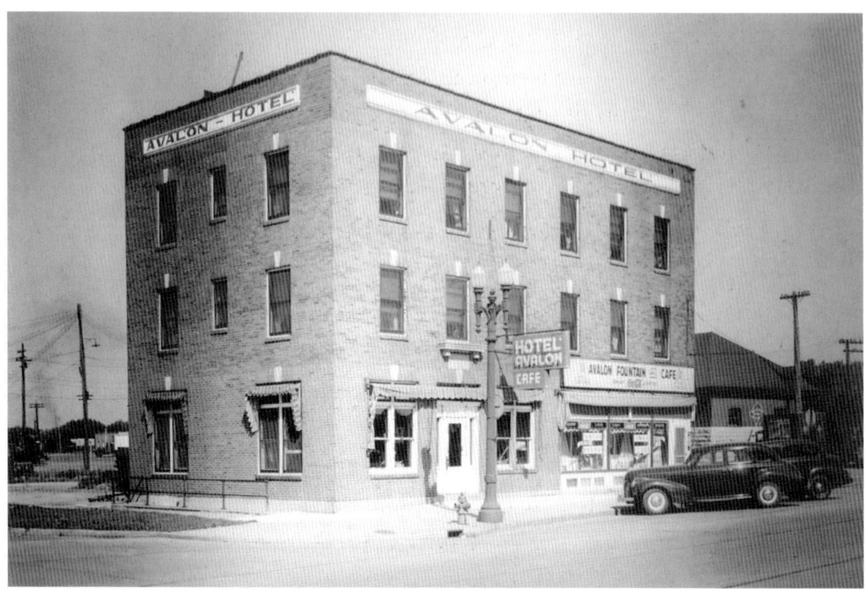

The Avalon Hotel. *Courtesy of the History Center of Olmsted County.*

be particularly progressive, socially or politically, in the pre–civil rights era. However, one day he reportedly walked by a bar on Third Street Northwest, on the north side of Central Park, and noticed a sign in the front window: "No N——s Allowed." He found it offensive. He entered the bar and asked for the owner. When the owner met him, after exchanging greetings, he told the owner that he did not like the sign and asked him to remove it. The owner declined. McQuillan then told the owner, "I'll give you a choice. You can take it down right now or I'll break your nose right now." The owner then complied promptly with his request. (Apocryphal story told to me by Walter Bateman and subsequently reported in the *Post Bulletin* by Mike Daugherty.)

Among my earliest memories as a preschooler growing up in Rochester is learning a racist version of Eeny-meeny-miny-moe and subsequently being told that the N-word was pejorative.

The first civil rights march held in Rochester was in August 1963. It included thirty-eight Rochester residents. They marched from Silver Lake Park to Soldiers Field Park. They were heckled and pelted with eggs by onlookers. That evening, a burning cross was placed in front of the Avalon Hotel by two eighteen-year-olds who were apprehended and fined. A subsequent editorial in the *Post Bulletin* stated in capital letters: "LET'S HAVE NO MORE CIVIL RIGHTS MARCHES IN ROCHESTER."[140]

In the 1960s, IBM was the first major business in town to recruit a more diverse workforce by hiring a small number of Black employees. Most lived in the northwest quadrant of the city, near the IBM plant. For that reason, their children attended John Marshall High School. I lived in southwest Rochester, so I attended Mayo High School. I was in the fifth class to graduate from the new school in 1971. There were over four hundred graduates per class. It was not until my class that the first Black student graduated from Mayo High School.

As Rochester has grown over the years, it has become somewhat more diverse. Toward that end, there has been some acknowledgement of Black heroes. The former East Park on East Center Street was renamed in honor of Dr. Martin Luther King Jr. in 2019.

George W. Gibbs Jr. Boulevard in Soldiers Field Park and George W. Gibbs Jr. Elementary School were both named in honor of George W. Gibbs Jr. in 2002 and 2008, respectively. Gibbs served in the U.S. Navy for twenty-four years, including duty as a gunner onboard a ship during World War II. In 1940, he served as a member of Rear Admiral Richard E. Byrd's third expedition to Antarctica, becoming the first Black person to set foot on Antarctica. Gibbs Point, located in Marguerite Bay on the Antarctic Peninsula, is named in his honor. He retired in 1959 as a chief petty officer. After earning a Bachelor of Science in education, Gibbs worked in the personnel department of IBM in Rochester from 1963 to 1982. In 1966, he was a founding member of the local chapter of the National Association for the Advancement of Colored People. After initially being rejected for membership in the Elks Club in Rochester, he integrated the club in 1974. He later served as president of the Rochester Kiwanis and the Rochester chapter of the University of Minnesota Alumni Association. After retiring from IBM, he founded an employment agency that he operated until 1999. He died on November 7, 2000, at the age of eighty-four and was survived by his wife, Joyce; two children; and one grandchild.

The recent history of immigrants moving into Rochester has been heavily influenced by wars, beginning with Indochinese immigrants after the war in Vietnam and Southeast Asia, continuing after the civil war in the former Yugoslavia and political instability and crime in Mexico and Central America. The influx of African immigrants accelerated during the civil war and famine in Somalia in the early 1990s. Minnesota has the largest Somali population in the United States. In 2000, the U.S. Census reported 1,131 Somalis in Rochester, out of 11,164 in the state, about 10 percent. According to the Minnesota State Demographic Center, in 2018, the Somali population in Minnesota was 33,500, second only to Mexico (64,500) among immigrants. (Other large groups include immigrants from India, 30,200; Laos, including Hmong, 24,400; Vietnam, 18,600; China, excluding Hong Kong and Taiwan, 18,600; Ethiopia, 21,900; and Thailand, including Hmong, 18,500. Estimates do not include United States–born children of immigrants.) Numbers are thought to underestimate immigrant populations because of trust and language issues. Estimates of the total Somali population in Minnesota range as high as 80,000.

Over the past forty to fifty years, the demographics of Rochester and Mayo Clinic have changed very substantially. Mayo Clinic changed from being a virtual white enclave when I started employment in 1984 to now having an international staff and receiving awards for diversity and inclusion. There is still progress to be made at Mayo Clinic and in Rochester as a community. Recent interest in Rochester focused on the Black Lives Matter campaign raises important questions that society as a whole and Rochester as a community need to deal with more effectively, strategically, humanely and generously. Mayo Clinic has made a substantial financial commitment to do so, and others in the community have spoken of the need to do likewise.

Mayo Brothers Commemorative Stamp, 1964

On September 11, 1964, the U.S. Postal Service issued a commemorative five-cent postage stamp in honor of the Mayo brothers, Dr. Will and Dr. Charlie. The issue was an acknowledgement of the centennial year of Mayo Clinic, dated from the arrival of their father, Dr. William Worrall Mayo, in Rochester in 1863 (or 1864 when his family joined him). The local

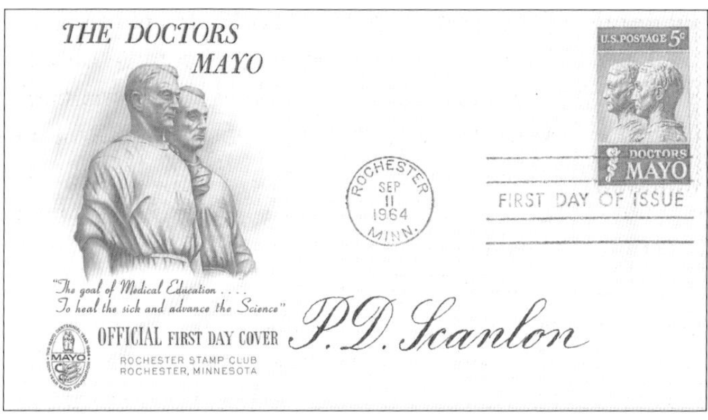

Mayo brothers 1964 commemorative stamp first day cover.

committee that advocated for the centennial stamp was chaired by Roy Watson Jr., president of Kahler Corporation. The stamp was designed by Victor S. McCloskey Jr. It included an image of the Mayo brothers based on the memorial statue by James Earle Fraser that stands in Mayo Park, as well as the words "U.S. Postage 5¢…Doctors Mayo" and an image of the staff of Asclepius, the Greco-Roman god of medicine. It was printed in green, considered symbolic of medicine. U.S. postmaster general John A. Gronouski spoke at a dedication ceremony in Rochester, calling the stamp "a tribute from a grateful nation for the good works of those men.…They left us a medical legacy of genius and generosity." A temporary postal substation was set up in the lobby of the Mayo Building to issue and cancel the stamps; 500,000 first day covers were handled that day. A total of 120 million of the stamps were printed.

LBJ

President Lyndon Baines Johnson and his wife, Lady Bird, were Mayo Clinic patients before, during and after his term as U.S. president. His first visit to Rochester was in 1941. The Johnsons were very popular guests at the Kahler and had many friends in Rochester.

On September 7, 1965, President Johnson, then fifty-seven years old, developed right upper-quadrant abdominal pain. He was suspected to have an inflamed gallbladder, which was confirmed by an X-ray procedure. He was also found to have a kidney stone in his right ureter. Mayo Clinic surgeon Dr. George Hallenbeck recommended surgery, which was scheduled for Friday, October 8, 1965, at Bethesda Naval Hospital in Bethesda, Maryland. Dr. Hollenbeck was assisted by Dr. Donald C. McIlrath, also a member of the Mayo surgical staff. The president chose a Friday to minimize the adverse impact on the stock market. The procedure was notable only for inflammation of the gallbladder. His operative course was unremarkable. The kidney stone was removed electively by Mayo Clinic urologist Dr. Ormand Culp through a small incision in the ureter. The procedure was completed in two hours. The president resumed his duties the next day and recovered uneventfully. Several days post-op, the president famously showed off his incision to the world. This was assumed by most to be an awkward photo-op at best. The president was cunning enough to know that the rumor mill would be buzzing with suspicions that his operation was for a more serious problem, such as cancer. He confirmed beforehand with Dr.

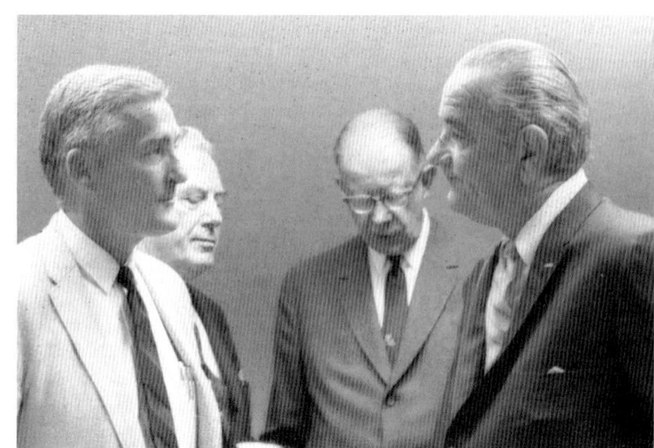

LBJ confers with Mayo Clinic Board of Governors chair L. Emmerson Ward at a 1969 Board of Trustees meeting. *By permission of Mayo Foundation for Medical Education and Research.*

Hallenbeck that a subcostal incision like his would never be used for a cancer exploration and his photo-op would thus quell the rumor mill.

President Johnson left office on January 20, 1969, and on February 21, 1969, began a four-year term as a member of the Mayo Clinic Board of Trustees. Sadly, he died of a heart attack on January 22, 1973.[141]

Benny's

During the summer afternoons and evenings of the 1960s and '70s, a very popular hot spot for Rochester teenagers was the R-tic Drive-in restaurant at the southeast corner of First Avenue and Sixth Street Southwest. It was better known as Benny's, after its owner, Benny Dresbach. Benny and his wife, Eloise, presided over the business and were well-known and well-liked by customers, many of whom were high school students. Customers could walk up or drive in, preferably the latter. Drive-in customers parked and were served by carhop waitresses who were chosen from popular high school girls. The specialties, and the only menu items most people remember, were root beer served in ice-cold glass mugs and Mexiburgers prepared with a secret recipe. It was a mixture of steamed loose ground beef lightly spiced and served on a white bread bun with ketchup, mustard, onions and pickle relish.

The highlight of the scene at Benny's occurred in 1965, when the Mustangs, a popular high school rock band, played a free concert for a crowd in the parking lot.

The Dresbachs operated the popular business from 1947 to 1978, when they retired and sold it. It remained open for several years under different owners. After it closed, it housed a sequence of small businesses. It was

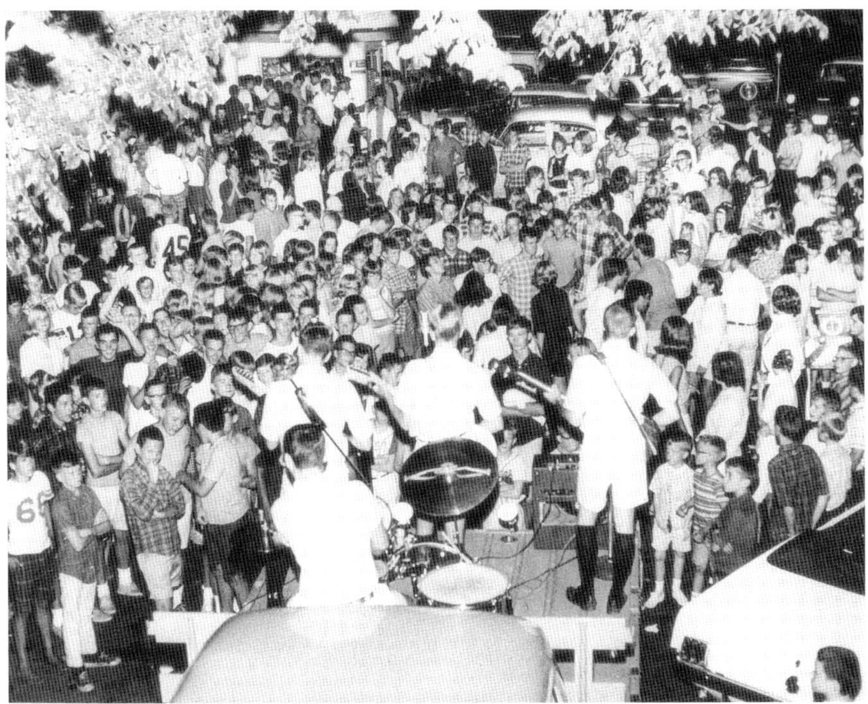

The Mustangs play an outdoor concert at Benny's. *Courtesy of the History Center of Olmsted County.*

eventually acquired by the neighboring VFW post and was then sold to the University of Minnesota–Rochester for campus development. Both were demolished on February 26, 2020.[142]

Solo Nobel Prize in Physics for Luis Alvarez, 1968

Luis Walter Alvarez moved to Rochester as a doctor's kid. His father, Walter C. Alvarez, was a gastroenterologist (GI specialist) at Mayo Clinic from 1926 to 1951. After Walter retired, he authored an internationally syndicated medical newspaper column and multiple books. The Alvarez family lived just over a block southwest of the Foundation House. Luis was born and had his early schooling in California. He was a bright student at Rochester High School, from which he graduated in 1928. He went on to a distinguished career that resulted in a Nobel Prize in Physics in 1968. Maybe even more remarkably, late in his career in 1980, he and his son Walter, a professor of earth and planetary science at University of California–Berkeley, published an article in *Science* from which the Alvarez Hypothesis derived.

Luis received his bachelor's degree, master's degree and PhD in physics from the University of Chicago. After graduation, he remained in Chicago. He made several important observations regarding nuclear structure and decay, including studies of tritium, the radioactive isotope of hydrogen. He described the use of Hg-198 (a naturally occurring isotope of mercury) for a reference frequency of light, used as a standard for precise measurements of distance.

In 1940, he moved to Boston to work at the MIT Radiation Laboratory, where he contributed to several World War II radar projects. Most importantly, he developed ground control radar, introduced in Britain in February 1943. This allowed pilots to land in zero visibility and was credited with saving many lives and many aircraft for the Allies late in the war and after. He also contributed to the development of transponders to distinguish friend from foe and an improved method for radar identification of enemy submarines. He created a microwave early warning system, as well as EAGLE, a precision microwave system for targeting bombs. EAGLE was used at the end of the war. It was more accurate under zero visibility than the Norden bombsight under clear skies.

After completing his radar and microwave work, he was assigned to the Manhattan Project. He spent a few months at the University of Chicago working on nuclear reactors with Enrico Fermi, and then he was reassigned to Los Alamos, New Mexico, with J. Robert Oppenheimer. His major contribution was the design of the implosion detonator for the plutonium bombs exploded in the Trinity test at Alamogordo and over Nagasaki. A subject of endless debate is the degree to which this device affected the Japanese decision to surrender. After the "Little Man," a uranium bomb, was dropped at Hiroshima on August 6, 1945, the Japanese showed no sign of surrender. They had the technology to detect that the bomb was a uranium bomb. They likely guessed, correctly, that we did not have enough fissile uranium (U-235) to build a second uranium bomb. Plutonium was more readily available than U-235, but a plutonium bomb is technically much more difficult to construct. When the Japanese realized that the "Fat Man," the Nagasaki bomb dropped on August 9, was a plutonium bomb, they would have known that we could continue building plutonium bombs. In fact, another was said to be available for use eight days after the Nagasaki mission. The Japanese surrendered on August 15, six days after the Nagasaki bombing. Alvarez addressed the ethics of President Truman's decision to use nuclear weapons in his autobiography. A more contemporary discussion is available in Chris Wallace's recent book *Countdown 1945*.

After the war, Alvarez served as director of the Berkeley particle physics lab. Under his leadership, the group developed a liquid hydrogen bubble chamber for observing subatomic particle interactions. They identified over half of the known subatomic particles. It was for this work that Alvarez received a rare solo Nobel Prize in Physics in 1968.

In 1980, Luis Alvarez authored, with his son Walter, a professor of earth and planetary science at UC–Berkeley, a paper in *Science* that is the basis of the Alvarez Hypothesis, the theory that the dinosaurs were killed by an asteroid impact sixty-five million years ago. Walter had observed a high concentration of iridium at the geologic boundary between the tertiary and the cretaceous layers of rock, the so-called K-T boundary. They hypothesized, with abundant evidence, that the iridium came from an extraterrestrial source, an asteroid.

Luis Alvarez is the only alumnus of Rochester Public Schools who has received a Nobel Prize. It could be argued that he deserved more than one. In 1998, when the Rochester School Board was debating the name for Century High School, I advocated, unsuccessfully, for naming it after Luis Alvarez.[143]

Notable Rochester Athletes

Herman J. Klinsmann was a bicycle racer. On July 15, 1893, he established the half-mile amateur world record of 1:06.5 on the horse racing track at the Rochester fairgrounds (now Soldiers Field). The following year, he established the professional record for the unpaced mile at 1:50.4 in Toledo, Ohio. He raced professionally for the E.C. Stearns team in 1894–96 until returning to Rochester to establish Klinsmann Co. (plumbing, heating, hardware, metal works and bicycles). He died in 1960, age eighty-nine, a lifelong Rochester resident.

Fred Fulton was known as the "Rochester Plasterer." Between 1913 and 1943, he fought 104 fights (83 wins, 72 by KO; 17 losses; 4 draws). In 2003, he was named to *Ring* magazine's list of one hundred greatest punchers of all time. He was six foot five and left-handed and had an arm span of eighty-four inches, a giant in his day. On July 27, 1918, he fought Jack Dempsey. He lasted only twenty-three seconds. He is ranked fourth-best heavyweight in Minnesota history by George Blair.

Roger Hagberg, running back, graduated from Rochester High School in 1957 and was named Minnesota State Athlete of the Year. He played for the University of Minnesota. He scored the winning touchdown against Iowa to send Minnesota to the Rose Bowl in 1961 (a loss to the Washington Huskies 17–7). He played four seasons with the Winnipeg Blue Bombers under Bud Grant and then five seasons for the Oakland Raiders under John Madden. With the Raiders, he played in 68 games and carried the ball for 194 rushes and 766 yards. In 1967, the Raiders were AFL Champions and played in Super Bowl II (1968), a loss to the Green Bay Packers (33–14). He was killed in an auto accident on April 15, 1970.

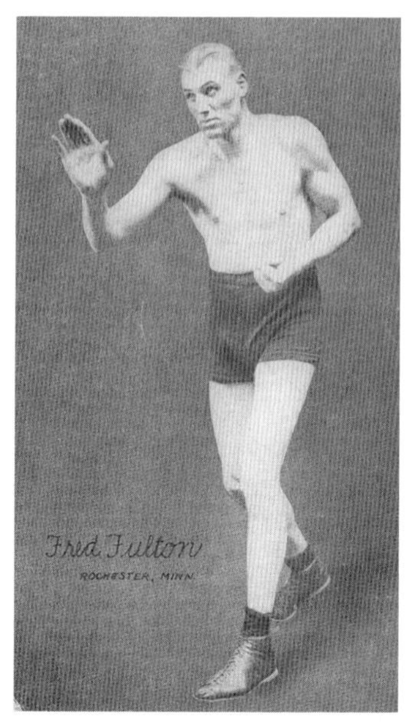

Postcard of Fred Fulton, boxer.

Pat "Irish" O'Connor was a light-heavyweight boxer, born in 1950. He won the 1967 Golden Gloves welterweight amateur national championship at age sixteen and fought his first professional fight at age eighteen with great fanfare. By 1972, he was undefeated at 31-0 and was expected to contend for a championship. In September, he was defeated unexpectedly by Andy Kendall. Thereafter, his style and good fortune deteriorated. He retired from boxing at age twenty-eight after three consecutive losses and was inducted into the Minnesota Boxing Hall of Fame. His career record was forty-seven bouts, forty-one wins, nineteen knockouts and six losses.

Mark Lutz graduated from Mayo High School in 1970. He was state track champion in the 100-, 220- and 440-yard sprints. The state records he established in each of those events were never beaten, and those distances are no longer contested, so they never will be beaten. He ran for the Kansas University Jayhawks from 1971 to 1974. In 1973, he won a gold medal at the World University Games in a 4x400-meter relay and was runner up at the USA Outdoor Track and Field Championships in 200 meters. In 1976, Lutz qualified for the Montreal Olympics in the 200-meter sprint. He was battling an injury and finished fifth in his qualifying heat. Mark was my teammate in basketball and track. He defined speed for many of us and was a great teammate.

Darrell Thompson graduated from John Marshall High School in 1986. After a stellar three-sport high school career, he played football for the University of Minnesota, where thirty years later he remains the all-time leader in career rushing yards, attempts, all-purpose yards and touchdowns, and he holds the record for longest run from scrimmage at 98 yards. He was the starting running back for four years and became the first Big Ten running back to rush for more than 1,000 yards as a freshman and as a sophomore. He was a Green Bay Packers first-round draft pick in 1990. In five seasons, he played in sixty games, gained 1,640 yards rushing and 330 yards receiving and scored eight touchdowns. He lives in Plymouth, Minnesota, with his wife, Stephanie Smith. They have four children who are all college athletes. He is the founder and president director of Bolder Options, a nonprofit youth mentoring organization.

Marcus Sherels was a return specialist for the Minnesota Vikings. A graduate of John Marshall High School, he excelled in football and basketball and rushed for over 1,000 yards in his senior year. He attended the University of Minnesota, where he qualified for a football scholarship as a walk-on athlete. In 2010, he was signed by the Vikings as an undrafted free agent. He is tied for first in Vikings franchise history with a 10.4-yard career punt return average (208 for 2,171 yards) and holds a Vikings career record with five punt returns for touchdowns.

Table 2
Other Rochester Athletes

Mark Brandenburg, tennis
Bruce Brown, diving
Rafael Butler, boxing and mixed martial arts
Eric Butorac, tennis
Tyler Cain, basketball
Phil DuBois, football
John Fina, football
Guy Gosselin, hockey
Sada Jacobson, fencing
John Johannson, hockey
Bruce Kimball, diving
Dick Kimball, diving coach
Bryce Lampman, hockey
Alec Majerus, skateboarding
Bethanie Mattek-Sands, tennis
Rocky McCaleb, boxing
Coco and Kelly Miller, basketball
David Morgan, golf
Leilani Muenter, auto racing
Scott Muller, canoeing
Joan Orvis, figure skating
Shjon Podein, hockey
John Pohl, hockey
Michael Restovich, baseball
Bob Schmidt, football
Scott Schneider, hockey

Howard Schoenfield, tennis
Aaron Senne, baseball
Jeff Siemon, football
Tommy Speer, mixed martial arts
Eric Strobel, hockey
Colin, Mark and Mike Stuart, hockey
Ben Utecht, football
Doug Zmolek, hockey

Many Rochester athletes have become professional athletes or have achieved other measures of greatness. Many of their achievements are memorialized in the Rochester Sports Hall of Fame by Rochester MN Sports (formerly Rochester Amateur Sports Commission).

Hotels—An Ocean Resort City with No Ocean?

When I was in college at the University of Minnesota, a classmate, who was a native of New Jersey, traveled to Rochester to interview for medical school. When he returned, he opined that downtown Rochester, with its numerous large hotels, reminded him of "an ocean resort city with no ocean." Since the turn of the last century, demand for accommodations

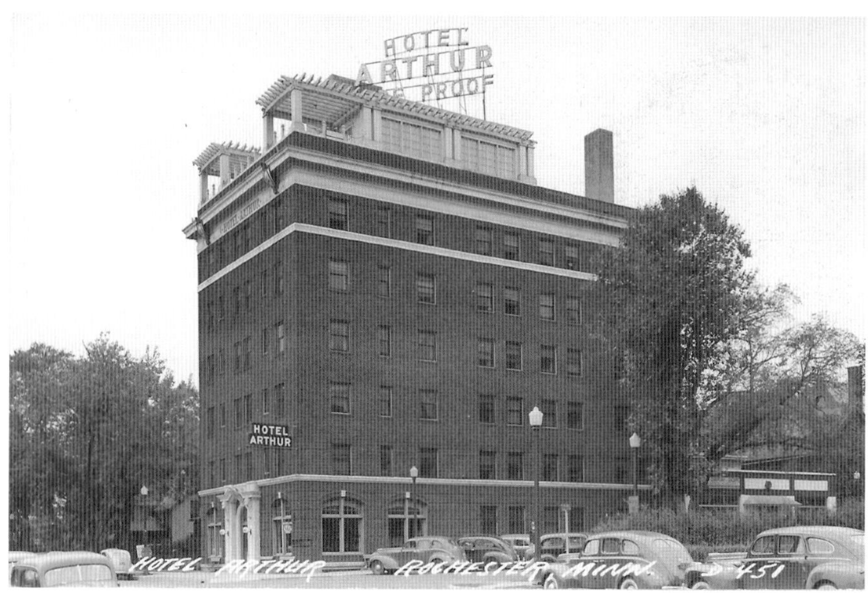

Postcard of Hotel Arthur.

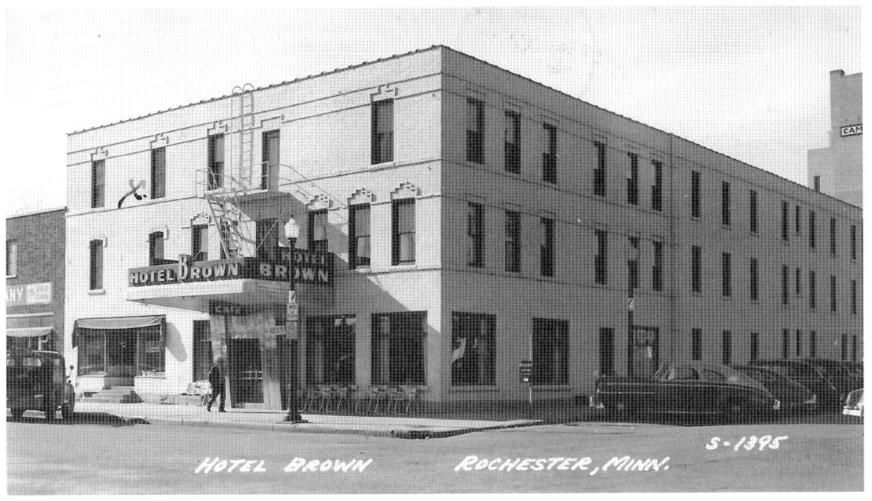

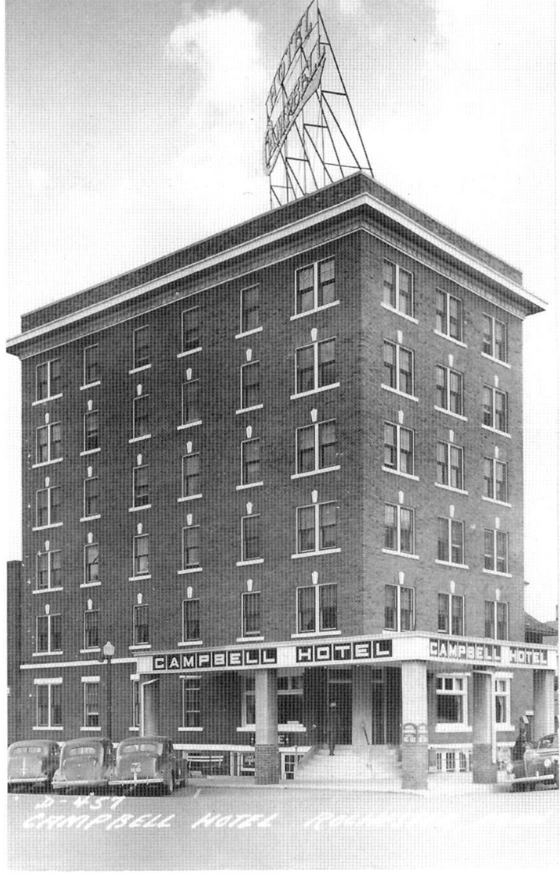

Above: Postcard of Hotel Brown.

Left: Postcard of Hotel Campbell.

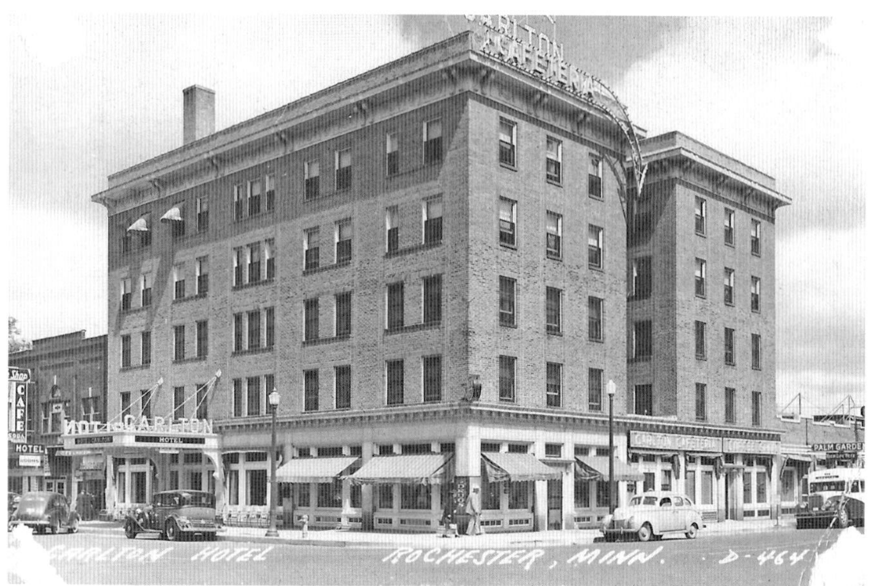

Postcard of Hotel Carlton.

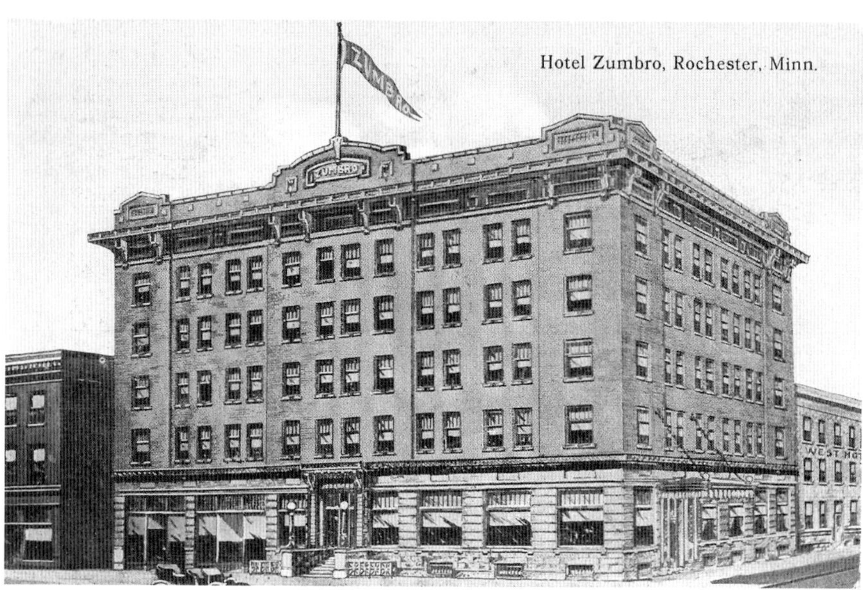

Postcard of Hotel Zumbro.

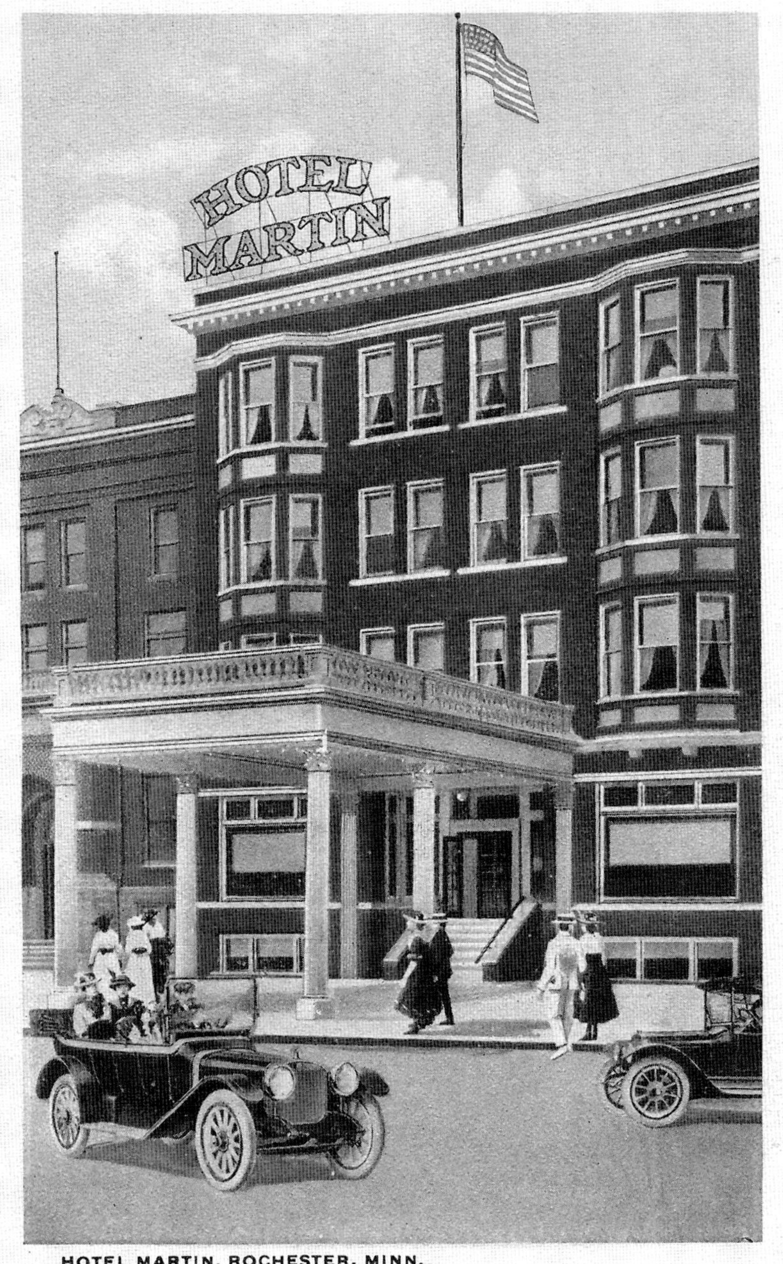

HOTEL MARTIN, ROCHESTER, MINN.

Postcard of Hotel Martin.

has often outpaced construction of new accommodations. A key to success for hotels in Rochester is filling beds on the weekends when the clinic is closed. That has driven recreational and cultural planning in Rochester with athletic events and cultural activities on weekends. The history of hotels in Rochester has been well described by Alan Calavano and Amy Jo Hahn.

The Flood of 1978

On July 6, 1978, I was in my first week of internship at Johns Hopkins. As I rode the morning shuttle to the hospital in East Baltimore, I heard several people in animated conversation discussing Rochester, Minnesota. I never expected to hear the name of my little hometown in such a location, so my ears perked up. What brought Rochester to national attention in the summer of 1978? The first television images I saw at the hospital were disorienting, showing a lake filling much of downtown Rochester.

The Zumbro River is prone to flooding. Floods have occurred over twenty times in the history of Rochester. The first recorded flood occurred on August 11, 1857.[144] Leonard mentions floods in the years 1859, 1866 and 1908. "The great freshet of 1882" was mentioned by the *Rochester Daily Bulletin* in reporting on the flood of June 23, 1908. The latter was memorialized with over forty different photographic postcard images. In more recent history, floods have occurred in 1925, 1942, 1951, 1962 and 1965. The flood of 1978 was the worst in terms of property damage and loss of life. In June, over five and a half inches of rain fell, saturating the region. On the evening of July 5, rainstorms moved through the region, dumping six to seven inches of rain overnight on Rochester and the Zumbro watershed south of town (estimated at over one billion cubic feet of water into the South Fork of the Zumbro and Cascade, Willow, Bear and Silver Creeks). The river began to rise rapidly, in places by over two feet per hour, prompting overnight evacuation efforts. Southeast Rochester was disproportionately affected because Bear Creek crested early at four o'clock in the morning. The Zumbro crested later at noon, eleven feet above flood stage. Four people died as a result of an elevator mishap in a nursing home, and one person died in Rock Dell Township. Heroic evacuation and rescue efforts by local law enforcement, plus the Rochester and Zumbrota National Guard units and volunteers, prevented more deaths. Over five thousand residents were evacuated. Property damage was estimated at $58 to $75 million. Clean-up efforts were massive.

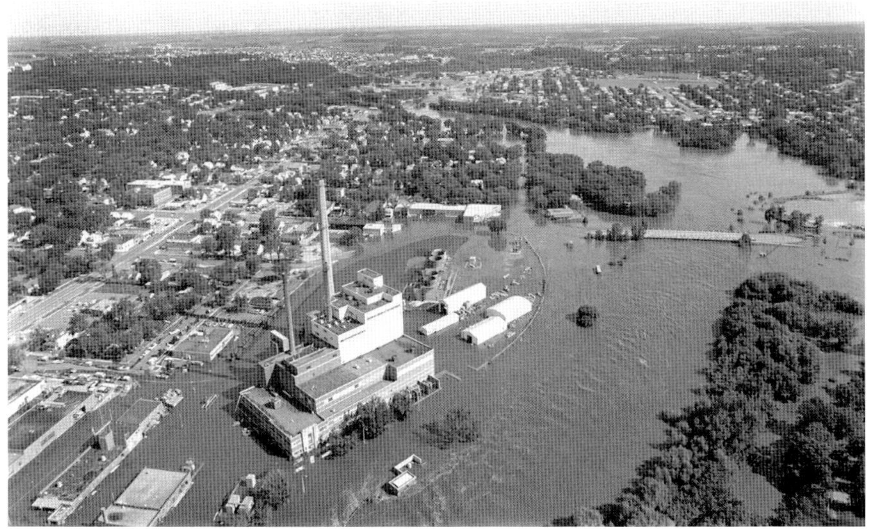

Aerial of flooded Rochester power plant bottom center, with Silver Lake to right, July 6, 1978. *Courtesy of* Post Bulletin.

Less severely damaging "100-year rainfall" events occurred in 1980 and 1981. In 1982 through 1987, city, county, state and federal funding sources were combined to fund the Rochester Flood Control Project. Construction began in September 1987 and was completed one month early, in August 1995. It was budgeted at $123 million but was finished under budget for $97 million. Included were upstream storm retention reservoirs (at Silver Creek, Chester Woods, Gamehaven, Willow Creek and three on Cascade Creek), channel improvements and bank stabilization through the city, thirteen pedestrian bridges and six and a half miles of bicycle and pedestrian trails with extensive bridge underpasses, plus river accesses, picnic shelters and canoe launches. Nineteen homes were removed from the floodplain. Additional local funds were approved to optimize the aesthetics, particularly through parks and downtown. The project converted what had been an unsightly river, formerly treated as little better than a sewer, into a continuous park through the city and through downtown. Since the project was completed, there has been no further flooding in the city of Rochester.[145] Bicycle paths have expanded outward and now total over eighty-five miles of dedicated park system paths (not counting on-street bikeways or Department of Natural Resources trails, for example, Douglas Trail).

Falcons, 1987

The peregrine (pilgrim) falcon is considered the world's fastest bird. When it stoops (dives for its prey), it reaches speeds exceeding two hundred miles per hour. In 1965, the peregrine falcon was endangered and nearly extinct east of the Rocky Mountains. This resulted from concentration of DDT in the food chain. DDT was a popular insecticide in the 1950s and '60s. It caused the falcons' eggs to be fragile by thinning their eggshells. DDT was banned in 1972, allowing falcons to begin to reproduce again, but their population was so diminished that they did not recover on their own. In the 1970s, attempts were made to reintroduce them in the wild. Owls are natural enemies of falcons and frustrated attempts to introduce falcons in rural areas. In 1977, a falcon called Scarlett was released by ornithologists from Cornell University at the U.S. Army's wildlife refuge on Carroll Island, Maryland, near Baltimore. She discovered the advantages of urban living for falcons: tall buildings that serve as surrogates of their native cliffs for nesting, great air currents around buildings, abundant populations of their favorite prey (pigeons) and lack of natural enemies, since owls avoid cities. She built a nest on the thirty-seven-story United States Fidelity & Guaranty Building (now called the Transamerica Tower) in downtown Baltimore.

Between 1979 and 1983, Scarlett was introduced to five captive-bred tiercel (male falcon) suitors, all unsuccessfully. Two were uninterested in breeding, one was shot, one was poisoned and one was hit by a car as he was recovering from a gunshot wound (a sad commentary on downtown Baltimore?). Despite her lack of success in breeding, Scarlett was an excellent single mom. Each year, she laid infertile eggs, which she incubated. After a thirty-six-day incubation period, scientists substituted healthy falcon chicks (called eyases), born in captivity, for her eggs. She successfully raised a total of eighteen adoptees. Finally, in 1983, a wild male, called Beauregard, began courting Scarlett. The following spring, the two mated successfully. They produced four eggs, which all hatched and were reared successfully. Sadly, Scarlett died that fall from an infection, but she had established the precedent of urban living for peregrines. Beauregard found a new mate almost immediately and sired another thirty-five offspring in the same downtown nesting site with two succeeding females. Since that success, falcon release programs have used tall urban buildings elsewhere for falcon release and breeding programs.

The Minnesota Falcon Restoration Project was a cooperative of the University of Minnesota's Bell Museum and the Raptor Center, the

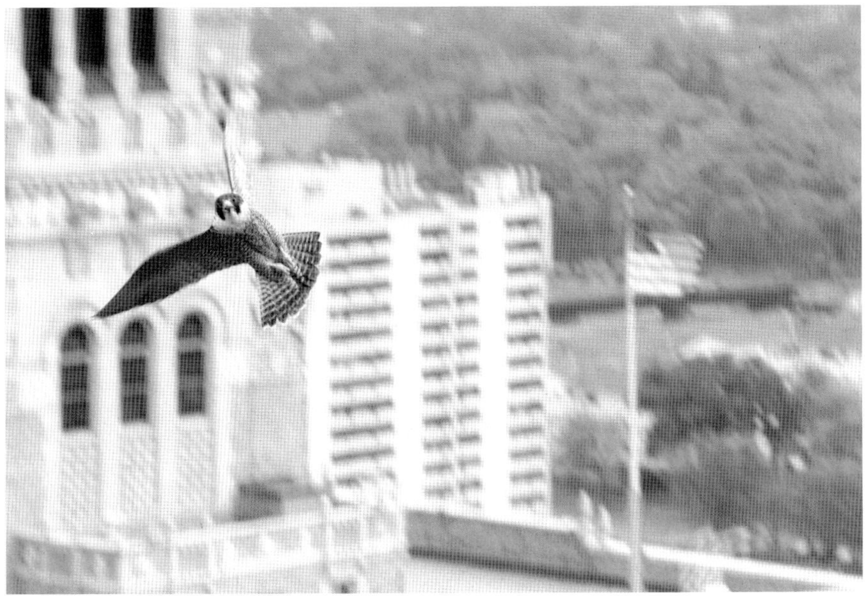

Peregrine falcon. *Courtesy of Jodi Jacobson.*

Minnesota Department of Natural Resources, the Minnesota Nongame Wildlife Program, the Nature Conservancy, the Midwest Peregrine Society and private falconers and breeders. The program was led by university ornithologist Harrison "Bud" Tordoff, who attributed his passion for falcons to his experience as a World War II jet fighter pilot. Beginning in 1982, the program used a method called hacking, in which chicks were hatched in captivity and then placed in nest boxes in favorable peregrine habitats. They were fed and cared for remotely by human attendants. At around forty days old, the chicks were allowed to fly free. This method of gradual release allowed the birds to adjust to life in the wild. Mayo's falcon program began in 1987. In its first two years, approximately eight chicks were raised each year in a hack box on top of the Plummer Building. The program was successful enough that hacking only continued for two years, after which returning falcons nested nearly every year, producing wild-bred offspring. The falcons quickly became self-sustaining. Falcons mate for life and generally return to a nest year after year. They have a high mortality in the wild, but if a falcon loses a mate, they generally, like Beauregard, return to the same nest and attract a new mate to begin breeding again.

Since 1989, a nesting box has been kept on top of the Plummer first, then Hilton and now Mayo. Video monitors follow the birds' progress as they incubate, hatch and mature. The eyases are usually banded and named in late May or early June. They fledge from the nest at about twelve weeks and spend the summer learning to fly and becoming independent. They migrate in the fall, but they occasionally return for brief visits in the winter. The parents defend their nesting site jealously, so only one nest can be placed in Rochester and the offspring need to find their own nesting sites. Over the years, falcons have provided great viewing for workers on upper floors of Mayo Clinic and other downtown buildings, soaring like little fighter planes. Seeing them dive to capture prey is a rare but thrilling sight. It is also fun seeing them up close when they land on the ledges outside the mirrored glass windows. As apex predators, they are not quiet and can often be heard screeching to each other from perches on the upper stories of downtown buildings.

Over the years, Mayo has had a successful breeding pair most years, usually raising two to four eyases per year. In 2018, Hattie and her mate, Orton, had four apparently healthy eyases. They all died suddenly in one day from inadvertent poisoning. In 2019, only one of four eggs hatched. That eyas was raised successfully. In 2020, the pair successfully fledged four chicks, three females and a male; however, two, Annabelle and Nadya, died from injuries, leaving Glory and Orville. Orton, the adult male, was injured in the summer of 2020 but recovered after treatment at the Raptor Center and was released in late summer back to the wild, where he reconnected with Hattie.[146] In the spring of 2021, the pair produced four eggs and shared incubating duty through late March and early April.

The Minnesota peregrine restoration program now produces 120 to 150 chicks every year. Since 1987, more than 2,500 wild peregrine chicks have fledged in Minnesota. Other Midwest states and Canadian provinces have followed Minnesota's example with similar success. The peregrine falcon was taken off the federal list of endangered species in 1999.[147]

The Brom Murders, 1988

In the early morning of February 18, 1988, sixteen-year-old David Brom, a high school sophomore at Lourdes High School, murdered his parents, Bernard and Paulette Brom, as well as his thirteen-year-old sister, Diane, and his eleven-year-old brother, Richard, in the upper level of their Cascade Township home. He delivered fifty-six blows with a twenty-eight-inch axe.

His victims were all in their pajamas when found. His older brother, Joe, was not living at home and was not involved. Later that day, David told a friend at Lourdes High School about the murder. He took the family's van but did not leave town. He slept in a culvert at a concrete plant that night. He was apprehended the following morning while making a telephone call at the post office.

The precipitating event was an argument with his father over a music album, of which his father did not approve. David had no prior history of violence or criminal behavior. He did have a personal history of depression, with two reported suicide attempts in 1987, and family history of mental illness reported by his grandmother. He was reportedly an "A student," and his schoolmates expressed incredulity at the crime, although it was reported that David had expressed his desire to kill his parents on multiple occasions, including the day before the event. His friends reportedly assumed he was joking.

David was tried as an adult and did not dispute any of the facts of the case but pled innocence by reason of insanity (McNaughten Rule). The insanity plea was rejected by the jury, and he was convicted on October 16, 1989, of four counts of first-degree murder. He was sentenced to three consecutive life sentences and one concurrent life sentence, a total of fifty-two years, making him eligible for parole in 2041, at age seventy. He is offender No. 146854 at the Minnesota Correctional Facility at Stillwater.

Blizzards

In 1872, William Worrall Mayo reportedly walked home from Kasson (eighteen miles), through the aftermath of a blizzard, when returning from St. Paul. He was too impatient to wait for train service to resume.[148] That is not the recommended approach to winter travel restrictions.

The National Weather Service reports records for snowfall. In Rochester, the record snowfall for a season was 86.8 inches in 2018–19; for a month, 41.3 inches in December 2010; for a day, 19.8 inches on March 18, 2005.[149]

One of the most infamous blizzards in Minnesota history was the Armistice Day Blizzard. November 11, 1940, started out as a beautiful, warm late fall day. Temperatures in the forties and fifties lured many out to enjoy the weather, particularly duck hunters. An understated weather forecast gave a "moderate cold wave warning." In the late morning, rain and winds began, temperatures

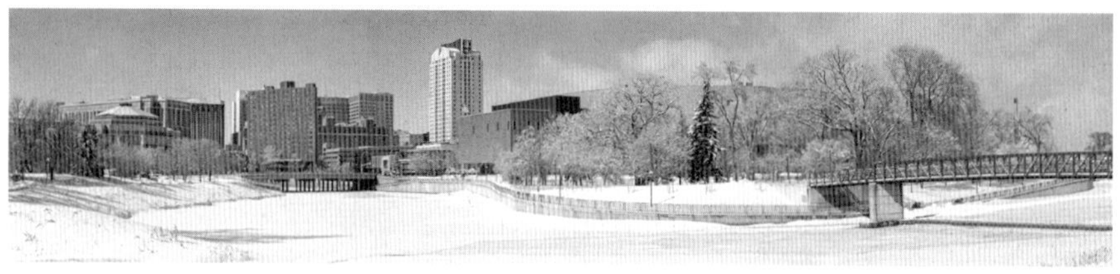

Panorama of Mayo Park, the Zumbro and downtown Rochester after a blizzard. *Courtesy of Dean Riggott Photography.*

plummeted and rain turned to sleet and then snow. The blizzard continued into the next day, with winds of fifty to eighty miles per hour, snowfall up to twenty-seven inches, snowdrifts up to twenty feet deep and temperature drops up to fifty degrees. The storm covered a huge area, including parts of Nebraska, South Dakota, Iowa, Minnesota, Wisconsin and Michigan. Nearly all roads were blocked, thousands of travelers were stuck and hundreds of duck hunters were endangered, many stranded overnight in terrible conditions. Communications were knocked out by fallen wires from the weight of ice and snow. A total of 146 deaths (49 in Minnesota) were attributed to the storm, including 66 people on boats on Lake Michigan and more than 20 duck hunters. In Minnesota, 1.5 million turkeys died. On November 7, the same storm had destroyed the Tacoma Narrows Bridge in Washington State (an incident familiar to most physics students).[150]

The Schoolhouse or School Children's Blizzard occurred on January 6–11, 1888. In similar fashion, it was preceded by unseasonably warm weather, followed by up to six inches of snow, high winds and extreme cold (negative fifty-eight degrees Fahrenheit in Neche, Dakota Territory; negative forty-seven degrees Fahrenheit in Fargo, Dakota Territory). It started on a school day, so many children became lost in the storm after being let out from rural schools. The result was 253 fatalities in the Dakota Territory, Nebraska, Iowa, Minnesota and Wisconsin.[151]

Many blizzards fill record books for the state.[152] Among the more memorable and more recent in Rochester history are the early season Halloween blizzard of 1991 and the late season blizzard of May 2, 2013.

Four days after the Twins won the 1991 World Series, the state was struck by a record early season storm, beginning on Halloween and extending through the next two days. Freezing rain, followed by snow, blanketed the region, knocking out power and communications, damaging countless trees and snarling up travel throughout the region. KROC News, in a retrospective article, said, "The precipitation total (rain and snow)

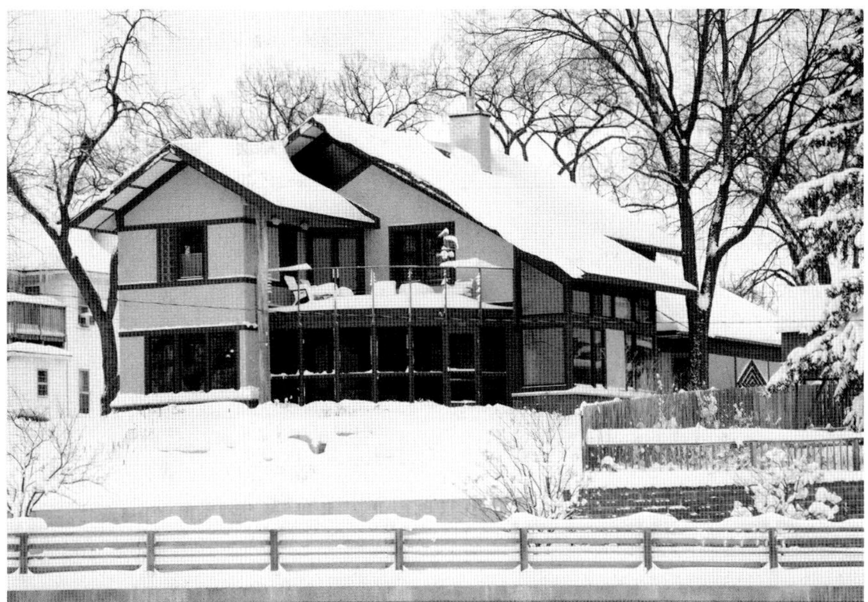

Blizzard aftermath.

recorded at the city airport was 2.3 inches, a daily record for the month of November that has not yet been broken. The snowfall total that day was 5.7 inches, one of the city's snowiest days for the month of November.…From 2–3" of ice accumulated across south central and southeast Minnesota.… Snowfall records were set elsewhere, all the way from the Twin Cities (28.4") to Duluth (36.9"—the largest single storm total in state history).… [A] 180 mile long stretch of interstate 90 from South Dakota border to Rochester was closed." Cleanup efforts were hindered by accidents and abandoned vehicles, as well as dangerously cold weather and winds of thirty to sixty miles per hour. Twenty Minnesotans died, mainly from heart attacks and traffic injuries.[153] Another large snowfall on November 29–30, 1991, added to the early season misery.

On May 2, 2013, warm weather yielded to plummeting temperatures and sticky wet snow that clung to everything, knocking down powerlines and countless trees and shrubs, bringing the city to a standstill. Ten thousand people lost power. A total of 14.3 inches of snow fell in Rochester on May 2–3, giving May 2 the fourth-greatest snowfall in the city's history. (In Dodge Center, 17.2 inches fell.) The snowfall for those two days was three times the total snowfall of all previous May snowstorms in Rochester history.[154]

Money Magazine—Best Place to Live

In 1993, *Money Magazine* ranked Rochester the number-one best place to live in America, among the three hundred largest metro areas. It continued to rank Rochester highly, with second place in 1994 and 1995 and third place in 1996. Rankings were based on top scores for health care, unsurprisingly, and transit (easy commute), as well as favorable scores for job market, low crime, quality of public education and relatively low cost of housing and property taxes. In 2019, *Money Magazine* ranked Rochester number fifteen in its top one hundred places to live. The article describing the ranking noted high-quality health care, long life expectancy, a strong job market, a short commute and cultural amenities. Currently, Livability.com ranks Rochester number five among its 2020 Top One Hundred Best Places to Live, after ranking it number one in 2016. The methodology of such rankings is suspect, and results are variable, but many in Rochester take pride in such plaudits.[155]

Barbara Woodward Lips

The Mayo Clinic Barbara Woodward Lips Patient Education Center is named in honor of one of Mayo Clinic's greatest benefactors. Mrs. Lips, from San Antonio, Texas, was a grateful Mayo Clinic patient for over forty years. She died at home on March 29, 1995, at the age of eighty-one. She left her entire estate, valued at $127.9 million, to Mayo Clinic.

She grew up poor, one of three children of a single mother in Durant, Oklahoma, during the Great Depression. She started her career as a lumber mill secretary in Oklahoma. Talented and ambitious, she worked her way up to a position in Dallas, where she met her husband, Charles Storch Lips, a ranching and oil magnate. When he died in 1970, they had no children, and she was only fifty-six. She actively managed their businesses for many years and amassed a much larger fortune as a widow. The estate included her home, plus thousands of acres of ranchland and oil and mineral rights in north Texas and Kansas. Her gift also included her fabulous collections of jewelry and antique furniture and decorative arts.

The gift, at the time, was the largest single gift to an educational institution in the history of American philanthropy, larger than Mayo's previous greatest gift from the estate of Mr. George Eisenberg. The gift is maintained in an

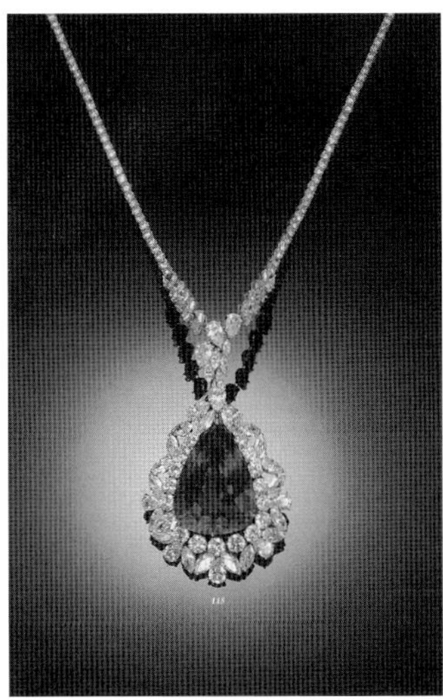

Barbara Woodward Lips's sapphire pendant. *Courtesy of Christies/Bridgeman Images.*

endowment with income used to support practice innovation, research and education. It came with very few constraints.

The jewelry was sold at auction by Christie's in a two-day auction in October 1995, the finest jewels on the first day and a collection of antique and period pieces two days later. Highlights included a diamond ring with a 51.24-carat European-cut solitaire diamond that sold for $596,500 and a sapphire and diamond necklace with a pear-shaped royal blue sapphire weighing 173.77 carats (42 millimeters by 31 millimeters) that sold for $420,500. The furniture and decorative arts, with estimated value of $800,000 to $1 million, were sold the day between the jewelry auctions. The auctions yielded a total of $7.7 million ($6.8 million after expenses). Several Tiffany lamps, a French vase and a music box were kept out of the auction for exhibit in the Mayo Foundation House.[156]

For comparison, the Hope Diamond weighs 45.52 carats. Mrs. Lips's brother said of the diamond ring, "She insisted on wearing it.... We didn't think it was safe, but we decided everyone would think it was glass, so she got away with it. She said, 'I didn't buy this to put in the safety deposit box.'"[157]

In addition to the Patient Education Center, the Barbara Woodward Lips Atrium in the Charlton Building is named in her honor. She specified a separate fund to provide a large fresh floral bouquet for Lips Atrium every week in perpetuity. The Charles Storch Lips Memorial Laboratory for Neurochemistry was named in honor of her husband in 1989.[158]

LGBTQI at Mayo, Oh My!, 2000

For much of my career, Mayo Clinic was a very in-the-closet place, where the gay and lesbian employees I knew were very selective about to whom they were "out." Undocumented, there were rumors of careers stifled or sidetracked because of revelations of sexual orientation. That changed suddenly in 2000. At a monthly administrative meeting with Robert Smoldt, who was then head of administration, Robert "Bob" Werner, a physical therapist, asked, "When will Mayo Clinic offer domestic partners benefits?" not expecting a positive response. Mr. Smoldt replied, "Beginning April 1." With a stroke of the administrative pen, Mayo became the largest employer in the state of Minnesota to provide domestic partner benefits, suddenly changing perceptions of Mayo Clinic and Rochester around the state. Since then, it has become a more gay-friendly environment. Although there is still room for improvement, Mayo Clinic Rochester now frequently receives awards and other recognitions for diversity, inclusion and equity.

ART AND HEALING—THE MAYO CLINIC ART COLLECTION

The 1914 Red Brick Building was built with a remarkable degree of architectural distinction, and the Plummer Building exceeded it in aesthetic detail. Both buildings can rightly be considered works of art, but neither included the explicit exhibition of art, per se, as part of its design or function. The Rookwood tile accents and Tiffany glass skylights were considered elements of craft as part of the 1914 Building design. The buildings did establish the rationale for the so-called "Healing Environment" of Mayo Clinic, however. Recall Dr. Leda Stacy's comment about the beauty of the building providing a "measure of peace and solace while awaiting their appointments."

The Plummer Building, built in 1926–28, was highly decorated with its Romanesque style, exterior of Indiana limestone, Italian terra-cotta accents, carved gargoyles, twenty-three-bell carillon, interior with carved stone, plaster-frieze ceilings, marble terrazzo floors and massive, ornate bronze doors. The purpose of that architectural distinction was well described by the internationally renowned architect Cesar Pelli, design architect of the Gonda Building. In a presentation to Mayo Clinic staff, he stated, "I envision Mayo's architecture as an important tool in the healing process....I wanted to design a building where the healing process begins the moment a patient enters the front door."

Although the buildings had beautiful aesthetics and the architecture might be considered art, the intentional placement of works of visual art did not occur until the construction of the new outpatient diagnostic building, subsequently called the Mayo Building, from 1950 to 1955. Plans for that building included the placement of commissioned murals in the lobby of each of its floors. The theme was titled "Mirror to Man." The initial ten floors were expanded to twenty in 1969. As part of the art program of the Mayo Building, bronze sculptures were commissioned for the exterior, including *Man & Freedom* by Croatian artist Ivan Mestrovic in 1954. The twenty-eight-foot-tall bronze figure has become the signature image of Mayo Clinic since then. In 2001, the Gonda Building was attached to the north face of the Mayo Building, where *Man & Freedom* was mounted. The statue was taken down, refinished with an interior patina and hung in the main atrium of the new building.

Since the initiation of the art program for the Mayo Building, placement of visual art, both two-dimensional and three-dimensional, has expanded greatly, to the point that there are now daily docent-led art tours at Mayo Clinic, available to patients, staff and visitors, as well as a self-guided audio tour. In addition to the benefits for patients and visitors, employees of the clinic derive pleasure and inspiration from the beautiful artworks. At a time when burnout is a serious concern for physicians and other health care workers, most Mayo employees would concur with the assertion that a beautiful workplace helps mitigate some of the emotional strain of caring for the sick on a tightly packed schedule.

Acquisition of art for placement in a facility such as Mayo Clinic must be done with great sensitivity. When budgets for research, education and care of the poor struggle to deal with life-and-death issues, expenditures for the arts may be seen as extravagant and subject to criticism. For that reason, much of the art placed in and around Mayo Clinic is supported by generous benefactors. Mayo Clinic accepts only a very few donated works of art, and only some of the most extraordinary works in the collection are donated in that manner. Many of the other works are commissioned as part of an organized art program and then subsequently supported by generous benefactors who provide the cost of the commission.

Selection, placement and curation of the artwork are the charge of the Department of Facilities. In the United States, there is a school of thought led by Roger Ulrich of Texas A&M University, who recommends a very limited style of art for placement in health care facilities. He asserts, from his research, that "results suggest a consistent pattern wherein the great majority of patients respond positively to representational nature art, but many react negatively to chaotic abstract art." Such works are called "healing art" by proponents.[159]

At Mayo Clinic, works such as those described by Ulrich are commonly placed in patient interaction areas, such as outpatient examination rooms and testing areas. Individually, these works are pretty pictures that might be quite nice and pacifying. Collectively, they can be boring and may not be of great artistic merit. In contrast, most of the artwork placed in public spaces in Mayo Clinic are more diverse, more contemporary and not necessarily representational.

As the art collection grew over the past sixty years, organization and management became a challenge. The design of the 2001 Gonda Building included an organized plan for placement of art because of its enormous size (1.5 million square feet). The art plan for the Gonda Building begins in the patient elevator lobbies, each of which has a display of ethnographic art from around the world. Emerging from the elevator lobby, a giant glass "wave wall" directs patients toward the main lobbies of each floor. Placed along the wave wall are one to three large works of glass art on each floor. They include works of many of the most prominent glass artists in the world. Each patient lobby has a thematic design with placement of the artwork around the large lobby. Works of art in the lobby are varied and include photography, selections of contemporary art and some sculptural pieces. Beyond the lobbies, in patient interaction rooms, visual images tend toward representational "Ulrich-style" works.

Works of art in the most public locations have the highest impact. The giant Chihuly glass chandeliers in the entrance of the Gonda Building have become the signature image of that structure. Thirteen externally lit chandeliers include 1,375 individual pieces of blown glass. Chihuly reportedly selected the color suite to be biological in appearance (yellows, greens and whites), reminiscent of the ocean. The bright, splashy colors are cartoon-like and provide a day brightener to patients and staff. The giant glass prisms by Stanislav Libensky and Jaroslava Brychtova sit in a quiet corner of the Gonda main level.

The bronze casting of *Jean D'Aire*, one of the Burghers of Calais, created by Auguste Rodin in 1884 to 1886, was a gift from a grateful patient. The pained expression on his face resonates with many patients and family members who are dealing with life-altering illness. It stands near Hage Atrium on the lower level of the Siebens Building. The collection includes other bronze works by Harry Bertoia, Douglas Olmsted Freeman, Harriet Whitney Frishmuth, Paul Granlund, Barbara Hepworth, Tuck Langlund, Carl Milles, Abbott Pattison, David Wynne and William Zorach.

Adjacent to *Jean D'Aire*, you can see one of the seven beautiful volumes of the St. John's Bible, a masterwork of calligraphy commissioned by the brothers of St. John's Abbey in Collegeville, Minnesota, and executed in

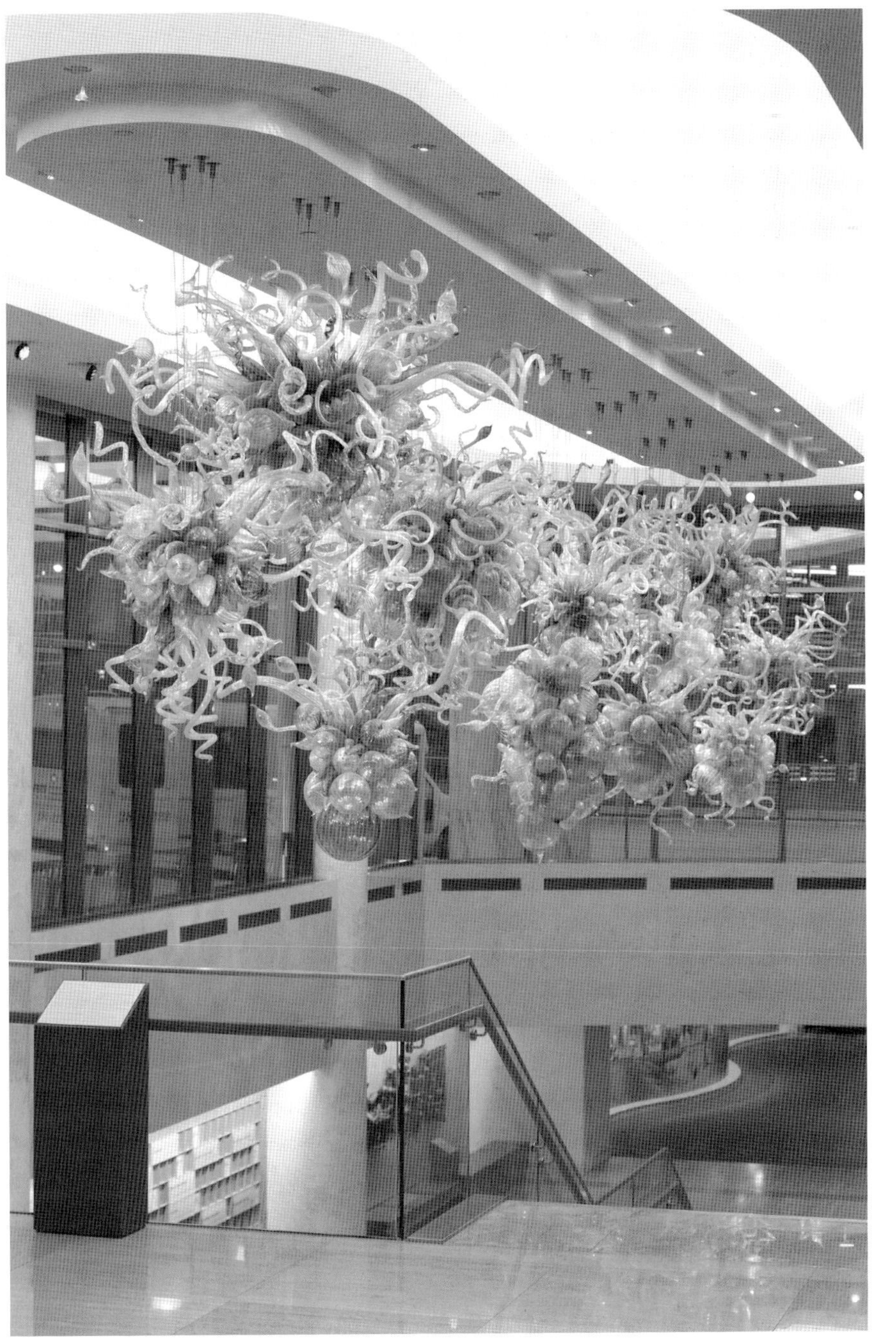

Chandeliers by Dale Chihuly in Gonda entrance. *By permission of Mayo Foundation for Medical Education and Research.*

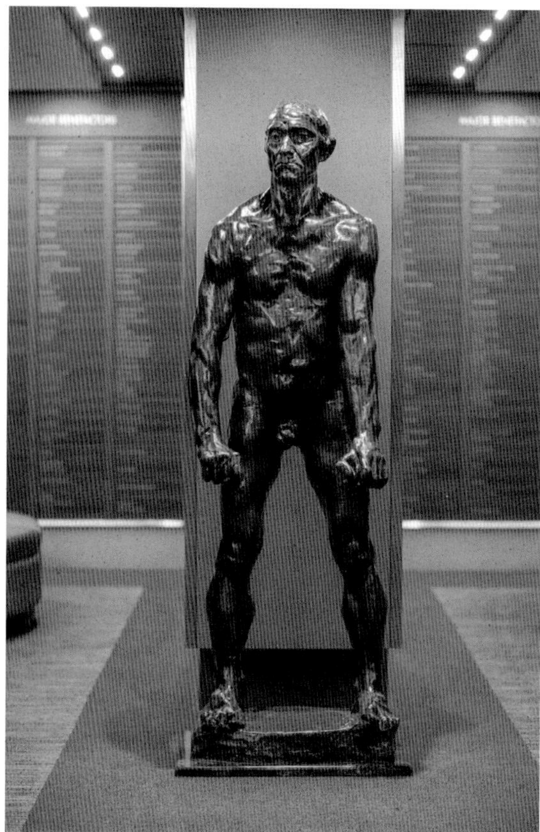

Jean d'Aire from the Burghers of Calais by Auguste Rodin. *By permission of Mayo Foundation for Medical Education and Research.*

Wales by Donald Jackson and his team of calligraphers and illustrators. Other volumes are displayed at Mayo Clinic Hospitals at St. Marys Campus; Methodist Campus; Jacksonville, Florida; Phoenix, Arizona; and Eau Claire, Wisconsin.

Fish, a mobile by Alexander Calder, hangs over the stairwell in the main lobby of the Mayo Building. It was a gift from Dr. Kaare Nygaard, a surgeon who trained at Mayo Clinic in the 1930s. He was an artist himself and a good friend of Calder, who inscribed the mobile to Dr. Nygaard. Other works by Calder provide primary colors and fanciful images.

A series of five giant lithographs by Joan Miró from the 1960s hangs in the patient lobby of the Hilton Building, which houses clinical laboratories. They, too, were a gift from grateful patients and are favorites among patients and staff. Their cartoon-like appearance and whimsical names (including *La Grande Ecaillère* and *The Big Oyster Woman*) bring a moment of levity to a very serious place.

Helen Levitt was a renowned New York photographer and a Mayo patient. One of her best-known photographs hangs in the Gonda Building's tenth-floor photography exhibit. (Coincidentally, the same image was printed with her *New York Times* obituary.) She was a friend and benefactor of Andy Warhol and collected his works. She gave Mayo Clinic ten images from his 1970 Flowers series, as well as ten signed images of the 1983 Endangered Species series.

The Israeli kinetic artist Yaacov Agam, a Mayo patient himself, has donated several of his works to Mayo Clinic, most notably his giant moving kinetic piece entitled *Welcome* from 1981. The pointillist *Four Houses* by New York artist Jennifer Bartlett hangs nearby in the Gonda lobby. A substantial collection of glass by Louis Comfort Tiffany is on display in various locations. One of Mayo's principal benefactors, Barbara Woodward Lips, amassed most of that collection. Other artists represented in the Mayo collection include Hans Arp, Henri Matisse, Jennifer Bartlett, George Braque, Jim Dine, Ellsworth Kelly, Jacob Lawrence, James Rosenquist, Robert Rauschenberg and Thurman Statom.

Mayo Clinic facilities in Florida and Arizona, which were founded in 1986 and 1987, have similar art programs, each supported by benefactors and bearing influences of local arts and culture. The art collection is described and extensively depicted in the book *Art & Healing at Mayo Clinic.*[160]

The art collection of Mayo Clinic serves the institution's primary mission, "the needs of the patient come first," by contributing to its Healing Environment. The collection, including the architecture, is artistically varied and maintains a museum level of quality. Contrary to some advocates, the collection includes modern and contemporary art, much of it abstract or non-representational. It serves as an institutional hallmark, providing healing, inspiration and entertainment for patients and visitors. For employees, it improves work experience and serves as a source of institutional pride; thus, it may reduce burnout and help maintain Mayo Clinic's remarkably low employee turnover.

Star Tribune: "Rochester Reelects Dead Man"

Dennis "Denny" Hanson was a member of the Rochester City Council, first elected in 1999 to represent the First Ward. Beginning in 2004, he served two four-year terms as president of the council. He was popular with citizens of the community, as well as the business community. On June 27, 2012, while running for reelection as council president, he died suddenly of a ruptured brain aneurysm at the age of fifty-seven. State law did not permit removing his name from the ballot in the November election or replacement with another name. His opponent, Jan Throndson, seemed destined for a shoo-in election. Hanson's campaign manager, John Eckerman, and his wife, Linda, and family felt otherwise. They expressed the desire to have a real election with two viable candidates. So, they continued to campaign for Denny to force a special election at a later date. Rochester responded by reelecting Hanson. Of forty-six thousand ballots cast, the vote was 51.5 percent for Hanson, 43 percent for Throndson and 5 percent for write-in challenger Jeff Thompson.

The response to this bizarre situation was surprisingly muted and dignified. Denny himself had a great sense of humor and would likely have gotten a good chuckle out of the situation. Randy Staver was appointed in July to serve as acting president in place of Hanson. He continued in that role after November. Throndson was good natured about the situation but chose not to run in the special election. Staver was eventually elected in a runoff on May 7, with Second Ward council member Michael Wojcik, although Wojcik had suspended his campaign a month earlier. Staver served as council president through two terms, until he chose not to run again in 2020.[161]

NATION'S BEST AND WORLD'S BEST MEDICAL CENTER

Since 1990, U.S. News & World Report has made annual rankings of the nation's best medical centers. Mayo Clinic in Rochester has consistently placed among the top three, most often number one, including the past five years (2016–20) consecutively. Mayo Clinic hospitals in Arizona and Florida rank as the best in their respective states.

Mayo Clinic in Rochester ranks among the top ten U.S. medical centers in fifteen of sixteen ranked specialties and has more number-one rankings (six) than any other center. Specialty rankings are based on expert opinion; patient survival; numbers of high-risk patients; hospital discharges; patient experience; nurse staffing ratios; availability of elite, highly trained subspecialists; advanced clinical technologies and procedures; certification for trauma care; professional recognition of physician and nursing staff (for example, Nurse Magnet status); and high performance in managing certain conditions and procedures. The 2020 specialty rankings include first place in diabetes and endocrinology, gastroenterology and GI surgery, gynecology, nephrology, pulmonology and lung surgery and urology; second place in cardiology and heart surgery and orthopedics; third place in cancer, ENT and rheumatology; fourth place in geriatrics; fifth place in psychiatry; sixth place in rehabilitation; and seventh place in neurology and neurosurgery. Mayo Clinic in Rochester is also ranked in eight pediatric specialties and ranks as the best pediatric hospital in the five-state region.

For the past three years, *Newsweek* has ranked the best hospitals in the world. Each year, Mayo Clinic has been ranked number one in the world.

Why Did They Build the World-Famous Mayo Clinic (the WFMC) in the Middle of the Cornfields in Rochester, Minnesota?

This is by far the most-asked question about Rochester and about Mayo Clinic. Helen Clapesattle began her book, *The Doctors Mayo*, with "The Paradox of Rochester," in which she noted the peculiar fact that one of the greatest medical centers in the world sits in a small town in the Midwest with little else to draw visitors from around the world. I believe a number of factors contribute to this curiosity:

1. William Worrall Mayo was the starting point. The father of the Mayo brothers emigrated from England in 1845. A restless fellow who was a tailor and a chemist by training, he traveled the American frontier, acquiring two medical degrees in the process. He came to Rochester as the examining physician for the Union army during the Civil War, with a letter of appointment from President Lincoln. After the war, he stayed in Rochester because his wife refused to move again. W.W. Mayo was a very skillful pioneer surgeon with great leadership skills that were recognized throughout Minnesota and beyond. He was a truly great mentor, not only to his sons. While they were young, he mentored several other rural Minnesota boys who showed intellect and initiative. One became an attorney who was Roosevelt's top trustbuster, president of the American Bar Association, U.S. senator, ambassador to Great Britain, U.S. secretary of state and Nobel Peace Prize laureate (Frank B. Kellogg). The other became one of the greatest entrepreneurs and philanthropists of all time (Henry S.

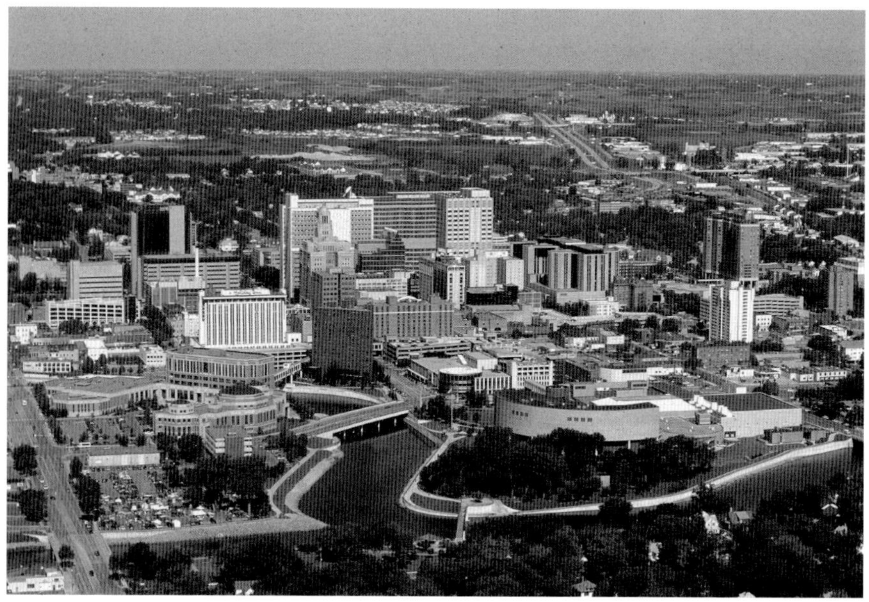

Aerial of downtown Rochester from the east. *Courtesy of Dean Riggott Photography.*

Wellcome). W.W. Mayo was also an activist for women health professionals (particularly Drs. Harriet Preston and Ida Clarke) and for the downtrodden, many decades before the world embraced his point of view. Lastly, together with Mother Alfred Moes, he founded St. Marys Hospital, which was the center of the Mayos' medical practice for twenty-five years before the first Mayo Clinic building.

2. Drs. William James and Charles Horace Mayo, the sons of W.W. Mayo, were great physicians and internationally renowned personalities during their lifetimes. Dr. Will Mayo, the older of the two brothers, declared shortly after his medical school graduation: "I expect to remain in Rochester and to become the greatest surgeon in the world." Few would express such confidence in a small town, but he was unwavering and succeeded in drawing the great leaders of medicine and the world to "beat a path to his doorstep." Harry Harwick wrote, "Doctor Will, a natural leader, was rather reserved, analytical, dominating (though without arrogance), relentless in demanding perfection of himself and others, with an uncanny ability to foresee the future."[162]

3. Dr. Charlie Mayo, Will's younger brother and complementary partner, had a very different personality, described by Harwick as "warm, understanding, wonderfully humorous, possessing the common touch."[163]

In a number of ways, Charlie was the more talented surgeon. He had a much broader range of expertise (ophthalmic surgery, ENT, neurosurgery, orthopedics, peripheral vascular and endocrine surgery), whereas Will concentrated on abdominal and gynecologic surgery. He was not nearly as outspoken as Will; in fact, he had to be persuaded to speak publicly. With effort, he developed an endearing style of speaking, very off handed with anecdotes and personal comments.

4. The Mayo brothers' careers coincided with a period of great opportunity in surgery. Dr. Will suggested to his biographer: "Stress the unusual opportunity that existed in the time, the place, the general setup, not to be duplicated now."[164] Given that the Mayos were great, what made their clinic great? That is, why did it last?

5. Unlike most academic medical centers, the Mayo practice, and hence Mayo Clinic, began as a clinical practice, with education and research following as second and third main missions. Of the three shields in the Mayo Clinic logo, the one that signifies clinical practice is slightly larger. In contrast, most academic medical centers begin with their educational mission first, with clinical practice and clinical practitioners in a subservient role. The mission statement, "The needs of the patient come first," is literally and historically true at Mayo Clinic and not elsewhere. It is not a coincidence that every Mayo Clinic employee knows and can repeat the mission statement and believes in it.

6. Although clinical practice has always had the dominant role, Mayo Clinic is a unique leader in post-graduate medical education. Mayo Clinic School of Graduate Medical Education is one of the largest, or perhaps the largest, and one of the oldest such programs in the world and has been since it began over one hundred years ago. Those who learned from the Mayos, both formally and informally, spread their teachings and their fame.

7. Teamwork has been an essential feature of practice at Mayo Clinic, beginning with the Mayo brothers. They were generous with support and praise for their teammates.

8. Specialization has been an early and enduring emphasis. The Mayos were always early adopters of new specialties as they first developed. With Henry Plummer and their team, they invented the multispecialty group practice. Practice innovation remains a high priority.

9. The allied health staff personify the Midwest work ethic, making for an extraordinarily productive workforce. In addition, they are empowered to lead and innovate. Countless examples reveal the benefits of such empowerment.

10. Will Mayo, Henry Plummer, Harry Harwick, George Granger and others created an innovative organization, a multispecialty group practice in a not-for-profit corporation with all-salaried professional staff, initially endowed by the Mayos' personal fortune. It is an extremely efficient model of medical practice and administration, even more so as the organization has grown. With great efficiency and enormous size comes great wealth, which can be directed toward institutional goals (practice innovation, research and education), thus creating greater opportunity for excellence.

11. The art of medicine is complementary to and additive with the science of medicine. The Healing Environment of Mayo Clinic includes the beautiful facilities and the cultural amenities they contain. Everyone who enters Mayo Clinic for the first time is struck with a sense of awe at seeing the gorgeous and enormous physical facility and all it contains. That experience is repetitively reinforced. Cesar Pelli, the architect who designed the Gonda Building, said, "I envision Mayo's architecture as an important tool in the healing process….I wanted to design a building where the healing process begins the moment a patient enters the front door." The Healing Environment is beneficial to patients and their families, as well as to staff and students.

Beyond the above factors, the analysis of the excellence of Mayo Clinic breaks down to thousands of data points and comparisons with the world's best medical centers. Those who make such comparisons consistently rank Mayo Clinic as the best, or among the best, both overall and in most areas of specialization.

So, the question is not "Why did they build the greatest medical center in an out-of-the-way place?" It should be, "Why did it become the greatest, despite being in such an unexpected small-venue location?" Rochester has grown with the clinic, so its history is inextricable from that of the clinic. I hope this book reveals some of the factors contributing to the successes of both Mayo Clinic and Rochester.

If Mayo is Rochester's bread and butter, it's also the knife, the plate, and the toaster.[165]

—Josh Noel

NOTES

Section 1

1. Eaton, *History of Winona*, 769–71.
2. Leonard, *History of Olmsted County*, 185.
3. Mitchell, *Geographical and Statistical History*, 111.
4. Leonard, *History of Olmsted County*, 189.
5. Ibid., 31–32.
6. Ibid., 25–26.
7. Bernard E. Sietman, *Field Guide to the Freshwater Mussels of Minnesota* (Saint Paul: Minnesota Department of Natural Resources, 2003).
8. Mann, *1491*.
9. Hamalainen, *Lakota America*, 253–55.
10. Eaton, *History of Winona*, 779.
11. Ibid., 862–63.
12. Leonard, *History of Olmsted County*, 283.
13. Mitchell, *Geographical and Statistical History*, 105.
14. Leonard, *History of Olmsted County*, 23.
15. Eaton, *History of Winona*, 637–39.
16. Raygor, *Rochester Story*, 45.
17. Hamalainen, *Lakota America*, 254.
18. Lincoln, "Message to the Senate."
19. Carley, *Sioux Uprising of 1862*.
20. Clapesattle, *Doctors Mayo*, 77–78.

21. Andreas, *Illustrated Historical Atlas*, 328.
22. Raygor, *Rochester Story*, 46–47.
23. John Weiss, "Sightings of Black Bears in SE Minnesota Increase," *Post Bulletin*, July 21, 2013.
24. Eaton, *History of Winona*, 772.
25. Mitchell, *Geographical and Statistical History*, 112.
26. Clapesattle, *Doctors Mayo*, 212.
27. Leonard, *History of Olmsted County*, 24.
28. Ibid., 281.
29. Severson, *Rochester*, 111.
30. "History of Log Cabin in Mayo Park," *Olmsted County Democrat*, September 7, 1906.
31. Mitchell, *Geographical and Statistical History*, 59–68.
32. Hartzell, *I Started All This*, 35.
33. Ibid., 142.
34. "Dr. W.W. Mayo Returns," *Olmsted County Democrat*, June 14, 1907.
35. Eaton, *History of Winona*, 731–32.
36. Code C.F. Mayo-Wellcome Relationships, correspondence to Alvin B. Hayles, August 9, 1976.
37. Mayo Clinic Historical Unit, MHU-0620 W.J. Mayo Correspondence, Box 104, Series 02/06/01, Folder F030.
38. Ibid.
39. "Owes Success to WW Mayo, Sir Henry Wellcome," *Post Bulletin*, October 18, 1935; Hartzell, *I Started All This*, 88–89; Anna E. Simmons, "A Company with Great Impact," *Science* 318, no. 5,853 (November 16, 2007): 1,071–73; "Garden City Dedication to Honor Onetime Pharmacist in Rochester," *Post Bulletin*, October 1, 1959; Mrs. J.W.B. Wellcome Jr., letter, "Memorandum of Some of the Activities of Sir Henry S. Wellcome (1853–1936)," November 12, 1946, the Mayo Foundation Library of Medicine, Rochester, Minnesota; William Hoffman, "The Long View from the Watonwan River," University of Minnesota Medical School, August 1995, https://www.mbbnet.umn.edu/hoff/hsw_art.htm.
40. Eaton, *History of Winona*, 790–91; Leonard, *History of Olmsted County*, 231.
41. Leonard, *History of Olmsted County*, 118–24; "Rochester State Hospital," MNopedia, Minnesota Historical Society, October 13, 2015, https://www.mnopedia.org/structure/rochester-state-hospital; Matthew Stolle, "No Longer Forgotten: Project Brings Patients' Stories to Life," *Post Bulletin*, October 14, 2016.
42. Eaton, *History of Winona*, 739–56.

43. Lee Morgan, "Spelunking in Minnesota," *USA Today*, April 25, 2020, https://traveltips.usatoday.com/spelunking-minnesota-60495.html.
44. Leonard, *History of Olmsted County*, 291.
45. N.H. Balaban, E. Calvin Alexander Jr. and Geri L. Maki, Geologic Atlas of Olmsted County, Minnesota, C-03, Plate 7, Sinkhole Probability, Minnesota Geological Survey, 1988, University of Minnesota Digital Conservancy, https://conservancy.umn.edu/handle/11299/58436.
46. Kim David, "Developer of Miracle Mile Project Seeks More City Assistance," Rochester's New-Talk KROC, September 6, 2017, https://krocnews.com.
47. Evans, *Cy Thomson*, 68–69.
48. Eaton, *History of Winona*, 741–51.
49. N.H. Balaban, Bruce M. Olsen, Geologic Atlas of Olmsted County, Minnesota, C-3, Plate 2, Bedrock Geology, Minnesota Geological Survey, 1988.

Section 2

50. Eaton, *History of Winona*, 757.
51. Leonard, *History of Olmsted County*, 140–50.
52. "August 21 1883 Rochester Tornado," National Weather Service, https://www.weather.gov.
53. Clapesattle, *Doctors Mayo*, 264–67.
54. Sister Joseph's node is an enlarged lymph node that can be felt adjacent to the umbilicus. It usually indicates advanced stage intra-abdominal malignancy.
55. Emily Carson, "Legacy of Mother Alfred Moes Continues to Guide Rochester Franciscan Sisters," *Med City Beat*, September 10, 2018.
56. Clapesattle, *Doctors Mayo*, 164.
57. Ibid., 177.
58. Harwick, *Forty-Four Years*, 5.
59. Mayo, *Mayo: The Story of My Family*, 24–27.
60. Clapesattle, *Doctors Mayo*, 209.
61. Collected Papers by the Staff of St. Marys Hospital, Mayo Clinic, Vol. 2, 1910, 557–66.
62. Transcript of "The Lost Oration," remarks of William J. Mayo, MD, to the Senate Committee on Education, Minnesota State Legislature, March 22, 1917, https://alumniassociation.mayo.edu.

63. Clapesattle, *Doctors Mayo*, 539–57.
64. Ibid., 698–99.
65. Mayo, *Mayo: The Story of My Family*, 80.
66. Curt Brown, "From Internment to Mayo Nursing," *Star Tribune*, September 6, 2020.
67. Hoyt Finnamore, "Celebrating Nurse Anesthetist Education—Alice Magaw (1860–1928): Mother of Anesthesia," Mayo Clinic, January 26, 2015, https://sharing.mayoclinic.org/2015/01/26/celebrating-nurse-anesthetist-education-alice-magaw-1860-1928-mother-of-anesthesia/?utm_campaign=search; A.A, Magaw, "Review of Over Fourteen Thousand Surgical Anæsthesias," *Surgery, Gynecology, and Obstetrics* 3, no. 6 (1906): 795–99.
68. "Saint Marys School of Nursing Alumni Association," Mayo Clinic, College of Medicine and Sciences, https://college.mayo.edu; "Methodist-Kahler School of Nursing Alumni Association," Mayo Clinic, College of Medicine and Sciences https://college.mayo.edu; "RCTC History," Rochester Community and Technical College, https://www.rctc.edu; "Nursing at Winona State," Winona State University–Rochester, https://www.winona.edu; "Nursing Department History," Winona State University–Rochester, https://www.winona.edu.
69. "Off the Beat: What Ever Happened to Royal Rochester?" *Post Bulletin*, September 27, 1991.
70. Personal communication with Wally Arnold, Med City Marathon founder.
71. Leonard, *History of Olmsted County*, 215–16.
72. Anne Halliwell, "50 Years of Beer at Schuster Brewing Company," Rochester Magazine, *Post Bulletin*, March 9, 2018.
73. Petersen, LaBrash and LaBrash, *History of the Rochester Fire Department.*
74. Jerry Reising, "Miracle Mile Shopping Center Grew out of Cornfield 35 Years Ago," *Post Bulletin*, October 31, 1987; Steven Landon, "3 Firms Found Negligent, Caused City's Worst Fire at Miracle Mile," *Post Bulletin*, December 3, 1974.
75. Greg Sellnow, "Tire Fire Smoldered for More Than a Year," *Post Bulletin*, August 2, 2006.
76. "Rochester Fire Department Has 134 Years of Vivid History," *Post Bulletin*, December 12, 2000.
77. Leonard, *History of Olmsted County*, 218–20; Hodgson, *Rochester: City of the Prairie*, 70–71.
78. Leonard, *History of Olmsted County*, 229.

79. Hahn, *Lost Rochester, Minnesota*, 128–29.
80. Nelson, *Mayo Roots*, 2–103.
81. Leonard, *History of Olmsted County*, 227–28, 696; Hahn, *Lost Rochester, Minnesota*, 127–33.
82. Leonard, *History of Olmsted County*, 247–48.
83. Clapesattle, *Doctors Mayo*, 131–32.
84. Wright-Peterson, *Women of Mayo Clinic*.
85. Ibid., 174.
86. Hayes SN, Noseworthy JH, Farrugia G, "A Structured Compensation Plan Results in Equitable Physician Compensation: A Single-Center Analysis," *Mayo Clinic Proceedings* January 1, 2020; 95: 35–41.
87. *Physicians of the Mayo Clinic*, 1,319–20; Wright-Peterson, *Women of Mayo Clinic*, 107–9, 170–73; Leda Stacy, "Twenty-Eight Years at the Mayo Clinic," unpublished memoir, 1957, courtesy of Mayo Clinic archives.
88. Clapesattle, *Doctors Mayo*, 479–80; Nelson, *Mayo Roots*, 88–89.
89. Stacy, "Twenty-Eight Years."
90. Clapesattle, *Doctors Mayo*, 529–35; Ellerbe, "Ellerbe Tradition," 15–16; Hahn, *Lost Rochester, Minnesota*, 53–56.
91. Clapesattle, *Doctors Mayo*, 692–93.
92. Amy Jo Hahn, "LandMarks; Rochester Armory, Olmsted County," *MN History Magazine*, Spring 2018,
93. Allsen, *Century of Elegance*, 110–15; "Plummer House History and Facts," City of Rochester Minnesota Website, https://www.rochestermn.gov.
94. Nelson, *Mayo Roots*, 90–93.
95. "Answer Man," *Post Bulletin*, April 15, 2012.
96. Andreas, *Illustrated Historical Atlas*, 115.
97. Tom Weber, "On the Street Where You Live," *Post Bulletin*, August 10, 1991.
98. Tom Weber, "A City on the Frontline of a Pandemic in 1918," *Rochester Magazine*, May 2020; Matthew Dacy, "Mayo Clinic's Response to the Pandemic: 1918," *Rochester Magazine*, May 2020; "History of 1918 Flu Pandemic," Centers for Disease Control and Prevention, https://www.cdc.gov; "Philadelphia Parade Exposes Thousands to Spanish Flu," History, https://www.history.com; Tokiko Watanabe and Yoshihiro Kawaoka, "Pathogenesis of the 1918 Pandemic Influenza Virus," *PLoS Pathogens* 7, no. 1 (January 2011),https://www.ncbi.nlm.nih.gov.
99. William G. Le duc, "Minnesota at the Crystal Palace Exhibition, New York, 1853," Minnesota Historical Society, http://collections.mnhs.org/MNHistoryMagazine/articles/1/v01i07p351-368.pdf.

100. Leonard, *History of Olmsted County*, 57.
101. Ibid., 57.
102. Severson, *Rochester*, 203–7.
103. Calavano, *Postcard History Series*, 10.
104. Collaborative Design Group, "Soldiers Field Park Master Plan Outline Prepared for the City of Rochester Board of Park Commissioners," November 2016, https://www.rochestermn.gov; Soldiers Field Veterans Memorial, https://soldiersfieldveteransmemorial.org.
105. Cindy Scott, "Lens on History: The First Kahler Hotel," *Post Bulletin*, March 17, 2015,
106. Clapesattle, *Doctors Mayo*, 596.
107. Chad Lewis and Larry Fisk, "Kahler Grand Hotel," *Minnesota Road Guide to Haunted Locations* (blog), https://ghost.hauntedhouses.com.
108. "Giant Crane Collapses," *Post Bulletin*, October 8, 1964; October 9, 1964; October 19, 1964.
109. Clark W. Nelson, "40th Anniversary of Rochester Methodist Hospital," *Mayo Clinic Proceedings* 69, no. 9 (1994): 2.
110. "The 1950 Nobel Prize in Physiology or Medicine," *Mayo Clinic Proceedings* 75, no. 12 (December 1, 2000): 1,232. https://www.mayoclinicproceedings.org.
111. Nobel Prize, https://www.nobelprize.org.
112. Lawrence P. Gooley, "Northern NY's Frank Billings Kellogg, Trust Buster," New York Almanack, April 15, 2013, https://www.newyorkalmanack.com.
113. Ellerbe, *Ellerbe Tradition*, 42–43; Grand Opening Brochure, October 26, 1927.
114. Ellerbe, *Ellerbe Tradition*, 41.
115. Alyssa Frank, "Mayo Family Owns KLER, Rochester's Second-Ever Radio Station," Mayo Clinic Laboratories, December 29, 2016, https://news.mayocliniclabs.com.
116. Mayo, *Mayo: Story of My Family*; "'Chuck' Mayo: Doctor, Citizen and Statesman," *Minneapolis Tribune*, July 29, 1968.
117. Personal communication from Austin Ferguson.
118. Nelson, *Mayo Roots*, 154–55.
119. Christopher Snowbeck, "Mayo's Next Maestro: As Health Care and Technology Merge, the New Chief Leads a Venerable Institution Through an Industry's Crossroads," *Star Tribune*, July 20, 2019.
120. Ellerbe, *Ellerbe Tradition*, 41–42; "Plummer Building," Society of Architectural Historians Archipedia, https://sah-archipedia.org.

121. "Ear of Corn Water Tower," Roadside America, https://www.roadsideamerica.com; "Keep Rochester's Corn Tower?" KIMT News, December 13, 2018, https://www.kimt.com; "Corn Water Tower," Atlas Obscura, https://www.atlasobscura.com; "County Reaches Deal That Will—Among Other Things—Preserve the Iconic Corn Water Tower," *Med City Beat*, 2019, https://www.medcitybeat.com.
122. Masson Copeland, *Pill Hill*, 257.
123. *Post Bulletin*, July 19, 2014.
124. Ibid.
125. Calavano, *Postcard History Series*, 10.
126. "Mitchell Student Center (Former Library)—Rochester MN," Living New Deal, https://livingnewdeal.org.
127. St. Mane, *Rochester, Minnesota*, 108.
128. Eckberg D.J., "Icon Under Fire: The Giant Canada Geese of Rochester, Minnesota," honors thesis, University of Minnesota, May 5, 2010; Molly Monk, "How a Minnesota Town Fell In and Out of Love with Its Ginormous Geese: Like Most Human-Fowl Relationships, It's Complicated," Atlas Obscura, February 13, 2020, https://www.atlasobscura.com.
129. *Rochester Magazine*, June 2020.
130. "Reaching New Heights: Secret Stories of the Mayo Clinic Aero Medical Unit," Mayo Clinic History and Heritage, http://history.mayoclinic.org/books-films/heritage-films/reaching-new-heights-secret-stories-of-the-mayo-clinic-aero-medical-unit.php.

Section 3

131. Francis Helminsky, "Law, Medicine, and Justice Blackmun," *Mayo Clinic Proceedings* 69, no. 7 (1994): 698–99.
132. Linda Greenhouse, "Justice Blackmun, Author of Abortion Right, Dies," *New York Times*, March 5, 1999.
133. Nan D. Hunter, "Justice Blackmun, Abortion, and the Myth of Medical Independence," *Brooklyn Law Review* 72 (2006): 147–97; Clark W. Nelson, "Harry A. Blackmun and Mayo," *Mayo Clinic Proceedings* 74, no. 5 (1999): 442.
134. "Rochester Profile," IBM, https://www.ibm.com; "Rochester Chronology," IBM, https://www.ibm.com; Elizabeth Baier, "'Stunned Silence' as IBM Breaks News to Rochester Employees," MPR News, March 7, 2013.

135. *Mayo Clinic and Another v. Mayo's Drug and Cosmetic, Inc.*, No. 38,380, Supreme Court of Minnesota, March 2, 1962, https://www.courtlistener.com.
136. Andreas, *An Illustrated Historical Atlas*, 328.
137. Leonard, *History of Olmsted County*, 119–22.
138. Ibid., 229.
139. "Legacy of the Avalon," *Post Bulletin*, January 22, 2011.
140. Ibid.
141. T.N. Pappas, "Politics and the President's Gallbladder," *Bulletin of the American College of Surgeons*, July 1, 2017; "The Truth about Lyndon Johnson's Gall Bladder Scar," *FDR's Deadly Secret* (blog), March 29, 2011, http://fdrsdeadlysecret.blogspot.com; "Answer Man: LBJ, Lady Bird Were Frequent Rochester Visitors," *Post Bulletin*, July 24, 2019.
142. Lee Hilgendorf, "Lens on History: JM Juniors Let 'er 'Rip' at R-Tic," *Post Bulletin*, July 12, 2016.
143. Alvarez, *Alvarez*; Alvarez L.W., Alvarez W., Asaro F. and Michel H.V., "Extraterrestrial Cause for the Cretaceous-Tertiary Extinction," *Science* 208, no. 4,448 (June 6, 1980): 1,095–1,108; Douglas Preston, "The Day the Earth Died," *New Yorker*, April 8, 2019.
144. Hodgson, *Rochester*, 11.
145. "Flood of Memories; Memories of Flood," Rochester Neighborhood Resource Center, 2004.
146. John Molseed, "Mayo Clinic Falcon Found Injured," *Post Bulletin*, July 11, 2020.
147. Jennifer Huizen, "A Highrise for Peregrines: The 37-Year Saga of Baltimore's Falcons Has Given Conservationists an Intimate Portrayal of the Species' Amazing Recovery," *Audubon*, June 12, 2015, https://www.audubon.org/news/a-highrise-peregrines; Carrol L. Henderson, "A Passion for Peregrines: How These Falcons Returned to the Skies of Minnesota," Minnesota Conservation Volunteer, March–April 2020, https://www.dnr.state.mn.us/mcvmagazine/issues/2020/mar-apr/peregrines.html.
148. Clapesattle, *Doctors Mayo*, 134.
149. National Weather Service, "Rochester Snowfall Records," https://www.weather.gov/arx/snow.rst.
150. Ben Welter, "Nov. 11, 1940: The Armistice Day Blizzard," *Star Tribune*, November 11, 2015.
151. "Schoolhouse Blizzard," Wikipedia, https://en.wikipedia.org/wiki/Schoolhouse_Blizzard.

152. "Famous Winter Storms," Minnesota Department of Natural Resources, https://www.dnr.state.mn.us.
153. "The Halloween Storm That Hit Rochester and Other Cities," KROC News, October 30, 2016, https://krocnews.com/the-halloween-storm-that-hit-rochester-and-other-cities/?utm_source=tsmclip&utm_medium=referral.
154. Christopher C. Burt, "The Phenomenal May Snowstorm of May 1–3, 2013," *WunderBlog* (blog), Weather Underground, May 4, 2013, https://www.wunderground.com.
155. Will Oremus, "Why the 'Best Places to Live' Usually Aren't," *Slate*, October 31, 2017, https://slate.com.
156. "Auction of Dazzling Jewelry Collection to Benefit Mayo," *Post Bulletin*, August 30, 1995; "Christie's Magnificent Jewels Sold to Benefit Mayo Foundation for Medical Education and Research, New York, Monday, October 23, 1995," auction program.
157. "Mayo Benefactor Once Was Poor," *Post Bulletin*, March 2, 1996.
158. "Texas Widow Leaves Mayo $127.9 Million," *Post Bulletin*, February 24, 1996.
159. R. Ulrich, X. Quan, et al., "The Role of the Physical Environment in the Hospital of the 21st Century: A Once in a Lifetime Opportunity," Report to the Center for Health Design for Designing the 21st Century Hospital Project, September 2004, https://www.healthdesign.org.
160. *Art & Healing at Mayo Clinic*, 2014, Mayo Foundation for Medical Education and Research.
161. Richard Meryhew, "Rochester Re-Elects Dead Man: City Council President Couldn't Be Taken Off City's Ballot," *Star Tribune*, November 7, 2012.
162. Harwick, *Forty-Four Years*, 5.
163. Ibid., 5
164. Clapesattle, *Doctors Mayo*, 279.
165. Josh Noel, "Reluctant Tourists: Mayo Clinic Makes Minnesota City a Magnet for Millions," *Chicago Tribune*, January 11, 2009.

Sources

Allsen, Ken. *A Century of Elegance: Ellerbe Residential Design in Rochester, Minnesota*. Minneapolis, MN: Ellerbe Beckett, 2009.

———. *Houses on the Hill: The Life and Architecture of Harold Crawford*. Kenyon, MN: Noah Publishing, 2003.

———. *Old College Street: The Historic Heart of Rochester, Minnesota*. Charleston, SC: The History Press, 2012.

Alvarez, Luis W. *Alvarez: Adventures of a Physicist*. New York: Basic Books, 1987.

Andreas, A.T. *An Illustrated Historical Atlas of the State of Minnesota*. Chicago: A.T. Andreas, 1874.

Calavano, Alan. *Postcard History Series: Rochester*. Charleston, SC: Arcadia Publishing, 2008.

Carley, Kenneth. *The Sioux Uprising of 1862*. St. Paul: Minnesota Historical Society, 1961.

Clapesattle, Helen. *The Doctors Mayo*. Minneapolis: University of Minnesota Press, 1941.

Eaton, Samuel William. *History of Winona and Olmsted Counties*. Chicago: H.H. Hill, 1883.

Ellerbe, Thomas F. *The Ellerbe Tradition: Seventy Years of Architecture & Engineering*. Bloomington, MN: Ellerbe Inc., 1980.

Evans, Eileen. *Cy Thomson: The Generous Embezzler*. Rochester, MN: The Printers, 2011.

Hahn, Amy Jo. *Lost Rochester, Minnesota*. Charleston, SC: The History Press, 2017.

Hamalainen, Pekka. *Lakota America.* New Haven, CT: Yale University Press, 2019.

Hartzell, Judith. *I Started All This: The Life of Dr. William Worrall Mayo.* Greenville, SC: Arvi Books, 2004.

Harwick, Harry J. *Forty-Four Years with the Mayo Clinic: 1908–1952.* Rochester, MN: Mayo Clinic, 1957.

Hodgson, Harriet W. *Rochester: City of the Prairie.* Northridge, CA: Windsor Publications, 1989.

Leonard, Joseph A. *History of Olmsted County, Minnesota.* Chicago: Goodspeed Historical Association, 1910.

Lincoln, Abraham. "Message to the Senate Responding to the Resolution Regarding Indian Barbarities in the State of Minnesota." December 11, 1862. American Presidency Project, University of California–Santa Barbara.

Mann, Charles C. *1491: New Revelations of the Americas Before Columbus.* New York: Vintage Books, 2006.

Masson Copeland, Helen. *Pill Hill: Growing Up with the Mayo Clinic.* Charlotte, NC: Heritage Letterpress, 2004.

Mayo, Dr. Charles W. *Mayo: The Story of My Family and My Career.* Garden City, NY: Doubleday, 1968.

Mitchell, W.H. *Geographical and Statistical History of the County of Olmsted, Together with a General View of the State of Minnesota, from Its Earliest Settlement to the Present Time.* Rochester, MN: Shaver & Eaton, 1866.

Nelson, Clark W. *Mayo Roots: Profiling the Origins of Mayo Clinic.* Rochester, MN: Mayo Foundation for Medical Education and Research, 1990.

Petersen, Minard, Betty LaBrash and Elmer LaBrash. *History of the Rochester Fire Department: 1866–2000.* Minneapolis: University of Minnesota Printing Services, 2000.

Physicians of the Mayo Clinic and the Mayo Foundation. Minneapolis: University of Minnesota Press, 1937.

Raygor, Mearl W. *The Rochester Story.* Rochester, MN: Schmidt Printing, 1976.

Severson, Harold. *Rochester: Mecca for Millions.* Rochester, MN: Marquette Bank & Trust, 1979.

St. Mane, Ted. *Rochester, Minnesota.* Charleston, SC: Arcadia Publishing, 2003.

Wright-Peterson, Virginia M. *Women of Mayo Clinic: The Founding Generation.* St. Paul: Minnesota Historical Society Press, 2016.

Index

E

F

G

H

I

J

K

L

M

N

O

P

He served as a consultant for important environmental issues, including asbestos hazards in Libby, Montana, and the Minnesota Taconite Workers Health Study of asbestos-related diseases. He taught regularly in the medical school, ICU, clinic and pulmonary function laboratory. He retired from clinical practice on November 13, 2019.

Scanlon was born at St. Marys Hospital. His Mayo Clinic medical record number starts with a 1. He has lived in Rochester all but nine years of his life. He is actively engaged in the community, having served as president of Rochester Public Schools Board of Directors, president of Rochester Montessori School Board of Directors, president of the Rochester Art Center Board, vice-president of the Rochester Civic Music Board and president of the Rochester Park Board. He and his wife, Maggie, a retired nurse, have three children, a computer guru and two nurses, and seven grandchildren. His hobbies include cycling, skiing, kayaking, arts and architecture, antiques and local politics. He is a collector of antiques and memorabilia, particularly books and postcards related to Rochester, Minnesota, and Mayo Clinic.

About the Author

Paul David Scanlon, MD FACP, FCCP, is professor emeritus of medicine in the Division of Pulmonary and Critical Care Medicine at Mayo Clinic, Rochester, Minnesota. He trained at the University of Minnesota (bachelor of arts in humanities, cum laude, 1975), Mayo Medical School (MD, 1978), Johns Hopkins (internal medicine, 1978–81) and Harvard (Pulmonary and Critical Care Medicine, 1981–84). He was a member of the staff of Mayo Clinic in Rochester for thirty-five years (1984–2019). He served as medical director of the Mayo Clinic Pulmonary Function Laboratories, the busiest such laboratory in North America, for thirty years (1988–2018). He was the founding medical director of the Mayo Clinic Pulmonary Clinical Research Unit (1994–2019). He was the medical director of the Mayo Clinic Dolores Jean Lavins Center for Humanities in Medicine (2003–18). He was a member of the Mayo Clinic Historical Committee for thirty years and served as committee chair in 2001–03. Scanlon is author or co-author of over one hundred peer-reviewed scientific articles, as well as book chapters and editorials and a popular book on pulmonary function interpretation, now in its fifth edition. He is the senior author of the original descriptions of the nonspecific pattern and the complex restrictive pattern, which were previously unrecognized and, together, account for 15 percent of all complete pulmonary function tests. He was a practicing clinician in pulmonary and critical care medicine and active in clinical trials of therapies for chronic obstructive pulmonary disease (COPD) and asthma, as well as studies of pulmonary physiology and new developments in pulmonary function testing.